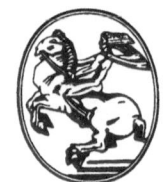

Topics in Infectious Diseases
Vol. 3

The Influenza Virus Hemagglutinin

Symposium, Baden near Vienna, March 21-23, 1977

Edited by
W. G. Laver, H. Bachmayer,
and R. Weil

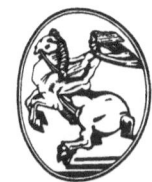

Springer Fachmedien Wiesbaden GmbH

The Influenza Virus Hemagglutinin
Sandoz-Symposium, Baden near Vienna, March 21—23, 1977

With 88 figures

Dr. William Graeme Laver
The John Curtin School of Medical Research,
Microbiology Department, Canberra City, Australia

Dr. Helmut Bachmayer
Dr. Rudolf Weil
Sandoz Forschungsinstitut Gesellschaft m. b. H.
Vienna, Austria

© 1978 by Springer-Verlag Wien

Originally published by Springer-Verlag Wien New York in 1978
Softcover reprint of the hardcover 1st edition 1978

Library of Congress Cataloging in Publication Data

Influenza Virus Hemagglutinin Symposium, Baden, Austria,
    1977.
    · The Influenza Virus Hemagglutinin Symposium, Baden
near Vienna, March 21-23, 1977.

    (Topics in infectious diseases ; v. 3)
    1. Influenza viruses--Congresses. 2. Hemagglutinin-
--Congresses. I. Laver, William Graeme,]929-
II. Bachmayer, Helmut, 1941-   III. Weil, Rudolf,
1932-   IV. Series.
QR201.I6I53   1977   77-17581

ISBN 978-3-7091-4132-8   ISBN 978-3-7091-4130-4 (eBook)
DOI 10.1007/978-3-7091-4130-4

INTRODUCTION

Influenza is still a major disease of man, regularly causing world-wide epidemics of varying severity which cannot be prevented by the vaccines currently available.

The main reason for our inability to control influenza lies in the extraordinary capacity of the two surface antigens of the virus - the hemagglutinin and the neuraminidase - to undergo antigenic variation.

Two kinds of variations occur in type A influenza, antigenic drift and major antigenic shifts. Variation of the hemagglutinin is of more importance than variation in the neuraminidase, since antibody to the former antigen neutralizes virus infectivity.

Antigenic drift probably occurs by the selection, in immune individuals, of mutant virus particles with altered antigenic determinants on the two surface proteins. These alterations are most likely caused by point mutations in the RNA and corresponding changes in amino acid sequences of the hemagglutinin and neuraminidase polypeptides. This mechanism, however, may not be responsible for the major antigenic shifts, and the new human pandemic influenza virus strains which arise from time to time may be formed by recombination between already well established human viruses and one of a large number of type A influenza viruses infecting animals or birds.

Over the past few years many new facts have emerged which may help us to understand the molecular mechanisms underlying the antigenic variability of the hemagglutinin. This molecule, which forms one of the "spikes" on the surface of the virus, is a triangular rod-shaped glycoprotein with a molecular weight of approximately 250,000. The hemagglutinin is synthesized as a single polypeptide chain which is glycosylated and cleaved during virus maturation into two smaller chains, HA_1 and HA_2, which remain covalently linked through disulfide bonds. Experiments with cross-linking reagents show that the hemagglutinin is composed of three HA_1 and three HA_2 subunits. The first results from sequence studies are now available which, if completed and extended to other hemagglutinin prototypes, could identify the changes in primary structure responsible for antigenic drift and antigenic shift. In addition, the development of methods to identify and isolate the hemagglutinin gene and to measure base sequence homologies between such genes provides a powerful tool for a novel genetic characterization of hemagglutinin molecules. Finally, new findings concerning the structure and biosynthesis of the carbohydrate moiety have shed some light on this specific modification of the precursor hemagglutinin.

These and other recent developments motivated us to convene the meeting in Baden in order to review the latest information available about the chemical structure of the hemagglutinin molecule and the relationships between structure, antigenicity and biological function of this unique viral protein.

Two other contributions which are related to these topics in a broader context, were also included in the program of the symposium: a discussion of some structural data concerning the fusion factor of Sendai virus which has some features in common with the hemagglutinin of influenza virus, and a general review of what is known about the chemistry of antigenic determinants on protein molecules.

It is hoped that the proceedings of this meeting will be of value to those who are working in the influenza field.

Perhaps in a few years from now, another Baden meeting will provide the answers to some of the unresolved problems of the influenza hemagglutinin.

The Editors

ACKNOWLEDGEMENTS

We would like to thank Academic Press, the Journal of General Virology, the Journal of Molecular Biology, the Journal of Virology and Virology for giving us permission to reproduce certain figures and tables in this publication.

Our thanks are also due to Miss R. Geisen and all those who ensured the smooth running of the meeting and to Mrs. A. Lembachner and Mrs. M. Taylor for their work on the preparation of the manuscripts.

We should like to acknowledge the partial support of this meeting provided by the Development and Applications Branch of the National Institute of Allergy and Infectious Diseases, National Institutes of Health, Bethesda, Maryland, U.S.A.

CONTENTS

X

XII

ANTIGENIC DETERMINANTS ON THE HEMAGGLUTININ SUBUNITS OF INFLUENZA A VIRUSES AND THEIR ROLE IN IMMUNITY

R. G. Webster and W. G. Laver

The hemagglutinin (HA) molecule of influenza virus is a glycoprotein of mol. wt. 210,000 and is composed of 3 subunits. The polypeptide chains making up each subunit may be cleaved or uncleaved depending on the host cell in which it was grown, in the cleaved state there are two glycopolypeptide chains HA_1 and HA_2 of mol. wt. 47,000 and 23,000, respectively (Schulze, 1975).

Antibodies to the hemagglutinin subunit are responsible for virus neutralization and are important in eliciting protection against infection. After infection or vaccination, antibodies are also produced to the carbohydrate moieties on the hemagglutinin subunit (Schulman, 1975). The hemagglutinin molecule shows antigenic drift when minor changes occur gradually within a family of strains. In addition, major antigenic changes (antigenic shifts) occur in the hemagglutinin molecule at 10-30 year intervals among the human strains. This paper deals with what is known about virus-specified antigenic determinants on the hemagglutinin molecule and their importance in antigenic variation and original antigenic sin.

Demonstration of Cross Reactivity and Specific Determinants on the Hemagglutinin Molecule

The number of different virus-specific antigenic determinants on the hemagglutinin molecule of influenza virus is not known (host specific determinants also exist on the hemagglutinin subunits). Recent experiments, however, have shown that the HA molecule of human influenza viruses possess at least two, and possibly more, virus coded antigenic determinants (Laver et al., 1974; Virelizier et al., 1974b). Thus, the HA molecule of influenza viruses within a major subtype, e.g., H3N2, possesses one or more 'cross reacting' antigenic determinants, and variants (A/Hong Kong/1/68, A/England/42/72, A/Port Chalmers/1/73) possess one or more 'specific' determinants. This is demonstrated in Table 1, with antisera to the isolated HA of A/Memphis/102/72 (H3N2) influenza virus prepared in rabbits. Absorption of the serum with A/Hong Kong/68 influenza virus removes all the antibodies reacting with this virus, leaving behind only antibodies to the specific antigenic determinants on Memphis/72. The antibodies dissociated from the Hong Kong/68 virus reacted with both the Hong Kong/68 and Memphis/72 strains, and are referred to as antibodies to the cross reacting antigenic determinants present on both viruses.

Immunodiffusion tests showed that the HK/68 subunits possessed at least two different kinds of antigenic determinants (Figure 1). One of the antigenic determinants was common to the hemagglutinin molecules of A/Hong Kong/68 and A/Memphis/102/72 viruses. Antibody to this determinant cross-reacted in immunodiffusion, hemagglutination-inhibition, and neutralization tests with

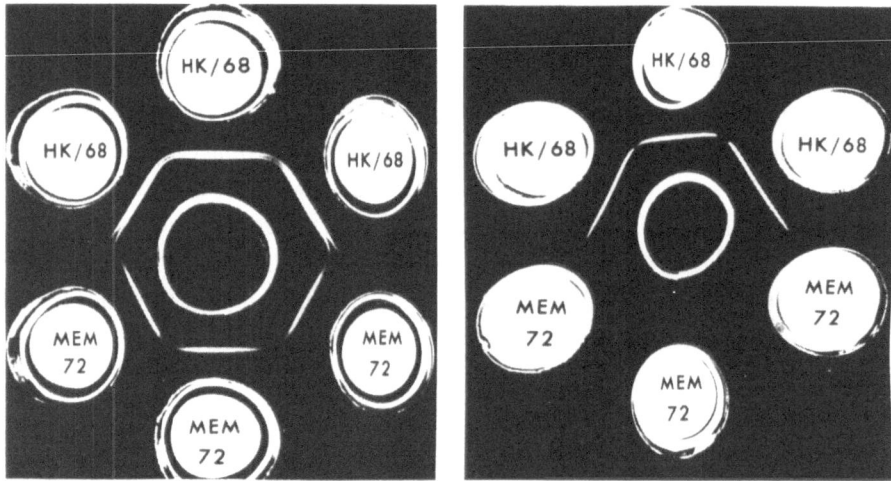

Figure 1
Double-immunodiffusion tests illustrating the preparation of antibody to the 'specific' antigenic determinants on the hemagglutinin subunits of HK/68 and Mem/73 viruses. On the left centre well, antiserum prepared against the isolated hemagglutinin subunits of HK/68 virus tested against particles of HK/68 and Mem/72 viruses disrupted with SDS, and on the right, centre well, the same antiserum after absorption with intact particles of Mem/72 virus. Absorption of the sera with the heterologous virus removed the antibody reacting with the 'cross reacting' determinant, leaving behind the antibody to the 'specific' determinant(s).

Table 1

Demonstration of Common and Specific Antibodies to the HA Subunits of Influenza Viruses by Absorption

Antisera to:	HI titers to the following influenza viruses		Kind of antibody present
	Memphis/72	Hong Kong/68	
Memphis/102/72 (H)	38,000	20,400	
Memphis/102/72 (H) absorbed with HK/68 virus	7,200	⟨50	'Specific' for Mem/72
Memphis/102/72 (H) dissociated from HK/68 virus	10,000	15,500	Cross reacting

Figures represent the reciprocal of the serum dilution inhibiting 3 out of 4 HI doses of antibody.

both viruses. Antibodies to another determinant showed no detectable sero-logical cross reactions between Hong Kong/68 and Memphis/72 viruses. Thus it appeared that during antigenic drift, Hong Kong influenza virus had under-gone a major antigenic change in this 'specific' determinant(s).

Location of the Antigenic Determinants on the Same Hemagglutinin Molecule

Experiments were done to determine if the different antigenic determinants were on different HA molecules or whether each molecule possessed a number of different antigenic determinants. ^{125}I-labelled subunits from Memphis/72 influenza were mixed with antibodies in the 'specific' or 'cross reacting' determinants of Hong Kong/68 and Memphis/72. Antibody to the 'specific' determinant on Memphis/72, to the 'cross reacting' determinant on Hong Kong/68 and to the 'cross reacting' determinant on Memphis/72 each precipitated the same amount of radioactivity as did unfractionated antisera to Memphis/72 hemagglutinin subunits (Table 2), indicating that the different antigenic deter-minants were located on the same molecule. Had the antigenic determinants been present on separate subunits, antibody to the 'specific' determinant should have precipitated only a portion of the labelled hemagglutinin.

Avidity of Antibodies to the 'Cross Reacting' and 'Specific' Determinant(s)

The antibodies were of high avidity for the homologous antigen, but reacted with very low avidity with the heterologous virus (Table 3). (The higher the value of K, the lower the avidity of the antibody).

Antibodies to the 'specific' determinant of Memphis/72 reacted to high affinity with the homologous virus. The antibodies dissociated from Hong Kong/68 influenza virus, – the cross reacting antibody population – reacted with high avidity with the homologous virus and with low affinity to the Hong Kong/68 strain. Thus, antigenic drift had occurred in the cross reacting determinant and a complete change had occurred in the specific determinant.

Diversity of the Antibody Response of Animals to the Antigenic Determinants on Influenza Viruses.

Antisera from different rabbits, hyperimmunized with HA subunits isolated from the A/Port Chalmers/73 (H3N2) strain of influenza virus, showed great differences in their 'cross reactions' with different strains of influcnza virus

Table 2

Precipitation of ^{125}I labelled Mem/72 HA Subunits with Antiserum to 'Specific' and 'Cross Reacting' Determinants

	^{125}I Labelled A/Memphis/72 B-HA			
	'Specific' HK/68	Unfractionated serum	Cross reacting HK + Mem/72	Specific Mem/72
Normal rabbit serum	+	+	+	+
	5%	68%	65%	68%
	5%			

100 μl of ^{125}I-labelled bromelain HA subunits from Mem/72 influenza virus were mixed with 5-40 μl of the above-mentioned antisera and allowed to react together for 60 min at 20°. Goat antiserum to rabbit α-globulin (50 μl) was mixed with the reaction mixture and allowed to precipitate at 4° for 16 hr. The precipitates were spun down and washed twice in phosphate-buffered saline. Additional washing did not further reduce the counts precipitated with normal rabbit serum. The figures represent the maximum amount of precipitation obtained in antibody excess. The residual counts not precipitated by the specific antiserum to HA were due to contaminating labelled neuraminidase known to be present and possibly other protein(s) liberated from the virus by bromelain.

Table 3

Avidity of Cross Reacting and Specific Antibodies to Influenza Viruses

	Avidity of antibodies (K) for:	
Antisera to:	Mem/72	Hong Kong/68
Mem/72 (H)	3.83	48.2
Mem/72 'Specific' (absorbed with HK/68)	6.82	No antibody
Mem/72 'cross reacting' (dissociated from HK/68)	6.03	20.5

The mean equilibrium constant (K) and the mean concentration of antibody molecules per milliliter were calculated according to Fazekas de St. Groth (1961). The larger the value of K, the lower the avidity of the antibody.

(Table 4). In HI tests, some sera reacted to about the same titer with A/Port Chalmers/73 and A/Hong Kong/68 viruses, suggesting that these two strains are closely related. Other sera, which reacted to high titer with A/Port Chalmers/73 virus, had only a low titer with the Hong Kong/68 strain, suggesting that the two viruses are distantly related (Laver et al., 1976). Evidence suggested that these diverse cross reactions were due to widely different ratios, in the different sera, of antibodies to the 'cross reacting' and the 'specific' antigenic determinants on the HA molecules. Thus, some rabbits gave a stronger response to the 'cross reacting' determinants than to the 'specific', whereas in others the reverse seemed to be the case. The selection of sera would greatly influence the designation of junior and senior strains of influenza virus. The results with antiserum number 2 (Table 4) would indicate that Port Chalmers/1/73 was senior to Hong Kong/68, but with the other antiserum these two strains could not be distinguished. These results show that it is important to select appropriate antisera for antigenic analysis of influenza virus strains.

Another important consideration is the time after immunization or infection. Early sera show few cross reactions with related viruses, but the avidity of the antisera increases with time after immunization, and so do the cross reactions (Webster, 1968).

The antigenic characteristics of the two groups of determinants of the hemagglutinin of A/PR/8/34 (H0N1) and A/FM/1/47 (H1N1) were investigated in inbred mice (Virelizier et al., 1974a,b). It was found that the antibody response to hemagglutinin was strongly dependent upon co-operation between thymus-

Table 4

Cross-Reactions of Hyperimmune Rabbit Antisera to the Isolated HA of
A/Port Chalmers/73 Influenza Virus

	HI titers to the following influenza viruses:	
Serum †	Port Chalmers/73	Hong Kong/68
1	24,000	16,000
2	32,000	480
1 (absorbed) ‡	12,000	‹10
2 (absorbed) ‡	32,000	‹10

†   Numbers 1 and 2 refer to single bleeds from different rabbits, collected 7 days after hyperimmunization.

‡   Serum absorbed with Hong Kong/68 influenza virus.

derived (T) lymphocytes and bone-marrow derived (B) lymphocytes. However, the dependence of the antibody response on the T cell for the 'cross reacting' determinant could be overcome by repeated immunization while induction of antibody to the 'specific' determinant was totally T-cell dependent. These findings indicated that the two portions of the hemagglutinin molecule were handled differently by the mouse immunological system. The studies of Virelizier et al. (1974a,b) also provided the possibility of examining the basis of antigenic memory for the hemagglutinin antigen and was found to be dependent on B lymphocytes and independent of T lymphocytes. These findings have important implications for the mechanism of 'original antigenic sin' for influenza which occurs when animals or man are exposed sequentially to two or more antigenically related hemagglutinins. The phenomenon of 'original antigenic sin' appears to be dependent on the antigenic memory of B lymphocytes but may be modulated by T lymphocytes (Virelizier et al., 1974b).

The Antibody Response of Man to the Different Antigenic Determinants on Influenza Viruses: Original Antigenic Sin.

The antibody response of man to the different antigenic determinants on influenza virus depends on the previous experience of the person with antigenically related influenza viruses. If the person has not previously been infected or vaccinated with the particular influenza subtype then he will produce an antibody response similar to that described above for unprimed animals. On the other hand, if man has been infected or vaccinated with a related strain of influenza virus, he will give an aberrant response. The antibody produced in response to re-infection or vaccination with a related strain of virus would be directed against the first invader. This recall of antibody to the first influenza virus experienced, by a related virus, has been aptly termed 'original antigenic sin' and has been studied extensively in humans and in experimental animals. (Francis *et al.*, 1953; Fazekas and Webster, 1966; Virelizier *et al.*, 1974b).

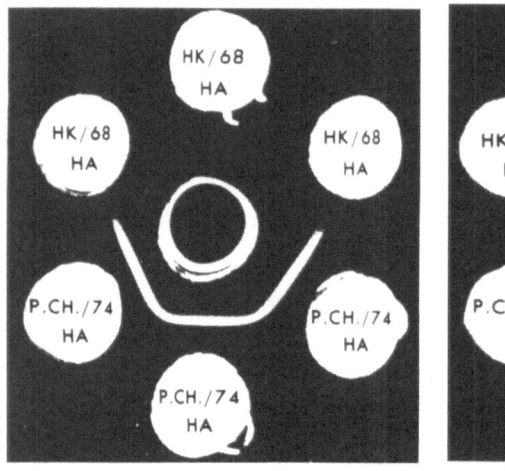

RABBIT SERUM IN CENTER   HUMAN SERUM IN CENTER

VACCINATION WITH PORT CHALMERS/74 HA

Figure 2

Double-immunodiffusion tests showing diversity in the immune response of rabbits and humans to A/Port Chalmers/73 hemagglutinin. The rabbit has responded mainly to the 'specific' antigenic determinants on Port Chalmers/73 hemagglutinin and the serum (left) contains antibodies which react preferentially with this virus. The human, on the other hand, has responded exclusively to the 'cross reacting, antigenic determinants on Port Chalmers/73 hemagglutinin subunits and the serum contains antibodies which react equally well with Hong Kong/68 and Port Chalmers/73 viruses.

These features are illustrated by double immunodiffusion (Figure 2); rabbit antiserum to A/Port Chalmers/73 gives a weak line of partial identity with A/Hong Kong/68 influenza indicated by a spur, while human serum shows a line of identity between the two viruses. The line of identity between the two viruses results from the recall of antibodies to the 'cross reacting' determinant. The response of human adults to influenza virus vaccines can be divided into four groups on the basis of adsorption characteristics (Table 5).

9

Table 5

Designation of Kinds of Antibodies Produced in Humans after Vaccination with A/Scotland/840/74 Influenza Virus.

Absorbing Virus	HI Titer after Absorption Hong Kong	Scotland	Designation of Predominant Antibody
Nil	6,100	2,500	
Hong Kong	<50	<50	Cross Reacting
Scotland	<50	<50	
Nil	8,500	2,200	
Hong Kong	<50	<50	Cross Reacting + 'Specific' Hong Kong
Scotland	1,100	<50	
Nil	5,100	4,500	
Hong Kong	<50	2,200	'Specific' Scotland + Cross Reacting
Scotland	<50	<50	
Nil	2,500	1,200	Cross Reacting +
Hong Kong	<20	300	'Specific' Hong Kong +
Scotland	500	<20	'Specific' Scotland

After immunization of human adults with A/Port Chalmers/73 influenza vaccine, the predominant kind of antibody response was against the 'cross reacting' determinants present on the HA of both Hong Kong/68 and Port Chalmers/73 (Table 6). Some individuals failed to produce specific antibodies to Port Chalmers/73, but paradoxically responded to the specific determinants on the HA of Hong Kong/68; others formed antibodies both to the specific determinants on the HA of Port Chalmers/73 and to the 'cross reacting and 'specific' determinants on Hong Kong/68 virus.

Table 6

Antibody Reactivity after Immunizing with A/Port Chalmers (H3N2) Vaccine

Animal	Kind of Antibody	Number
Rabbit	Cross reacting + Port Ch. Specific	6/6
Human †	Cross reacting	2/43
Human	Cross reacting + HK Specific	27/43
Human	Cross reacting + HK Specific + Port Ch. Specific	11/43
Human	Cross reacting + Port Ch. Specific	3/43

† All people were seronegative before vaccination.

The immune status of the subjects at the time of vaccination with Port Chalmers/73 seemed to be important, since the only people giving true primary response were two who had no detectable levels of antibody to Hong Kong/68. The majority of subjects gave a high antibody response to the common determinants present on both viruses. This is not surprising. What is surprising, however, is that most of these subjects, after vaccination with Port Chalmers/73 vaccine, gave a response to the specific determinants on the HA of Hong Kong/68, but no detectable response to the specific determinants on the HA of Port Chalmers/73. Studies in mice (Virelizier *et al.*, 1974b) have shown that, after sequential immunization with the HA of two related influenza viruses, a similar paradox occurred; some of the antibodies were directed to determinants present only on the first HA encountered.

Both of these responses are characteristic of the 'original antigenic sin' phenomenon after infection or vaccination with influenza viruses (Fazekas de St. Groth and Webster, 1966; Francis *et al.*, 1953; Virelizier *et al.*, 1974a,b). Studies on original antigenic sin to influenza virus can now be interpreted in terms of a diverse response to different antigenic determinants.

Efficacy of Antibody 'Type' for Protection of Man against Challenge with Influenza Virus.

Two practical questions arise from the above studies; what is the relative efficacy of the antibodies to the 'cross reacting' and 'specific' determinants in protection and is it necessary to change the vaccine formulation each time a minor antigenic variant becomes dominant. Studies in humans indicate that both cross reacting and specific antibodies will protect people from infection with influenza virus (Table 7), but higher levels of cross reacting antibodies are required to give protection. If low levels of cross reacting antibody are induced after vaccination, the volunteers could be infected and show clinical signs of influenza. On the other hand, volunteers who produced low levels of specific antibodies in addition to the cross reacting antibodies, shed virus after challenge for 1-2 days but showed no signs of illness. Thus antibodies to the 'specific' determinants are more efficient at giving protection from challenge with influenza virus, confirming the epidemiological evidence that incorporation of the most recent influenza variant in vaccines is necessary to induce protection.

Discussion and Summary

Antibody absorption studies have demonstrated that there are at least two different virus specified antigenic determinants on the hemagglutinin molecule of influenza A viruses. There are referred to as the 'cross reacting' and 'specific' antigenic determinants. The multiple antigenic determinants are located on each hemagglutinin molecule. During antigenic drift in a family of influenza A viruses, antigenic changes occur in both the 'cross reacting' and 'specific' determinants on the hemagglutinin molecule; the 'cross reacting' determinant retains antigenic similarity with the preceding strain while the 'specific' determinant on the new strain is serologically distinct from the preceding strain.

After immunization or infection, non-primed animals produce antibodies to each determinant on the hemagglutinin molecule of influenza virus. If the animal (or human) had been exposed to one strain of influenza and was subsequently infected or vaccinated with a serologically related strain an aberrant antibody response ensues. Thus, antibodies were induced to the 'cross reacting' and 'specific' determinants on the hemagglutinin molecule of the virus first experienced. Studies in man showed that antibodies to the 'specific' antigenic determinant(s) are more effective than 'cross reacting' antibodies at eliciting

Table 7

Efficacy of Antibody 'Type' for Protection of Man against Challenge with Influenza Virus

Antibody 'type'	Virus Isolation	Illness	HI Antibody Titer HK/68	Scot/74	Number of Patients
Cross reacting	+	+	150	40	
Cross reacting	+	+	130	60	
Cross reacting	+	+	160	300	6
Cross reacting	+	0	180	65	
Cross reacting	0	+	160	110	
Cross reacting	0	+	240	60	
Cross reacting + Specific	+	0	260	150	
Cross reacting + Specific	+	0	600	300	2
Cross reacting	0	0	$\geq$500	$\geq$120	11
Cross reacting + Specific	0	0	$\geq$1000	$\geq$360	12

Adult volunteers were immunized with A/Scotland/74 inactivated vaccines and challenged 47 days later with infectious A/Scotland/74 virus.

protection from infection. Antibodies to the 'cross reacting' determinants will provide protection, providing there are high levels of antibody present.

The aberrant response or the recall of antibodies to the determinants on one influenza A virus after exposure to another influenza virus in that family, is characteristic of 'original antigenic sin'. The question of how a 'specific' determinant (S2) can recall antibodies to the 'specific' determinant (S1) on an earlier strain is difficult to explain, since antibody to S1 does not react with S2 in serological tests.

One explanation for this may be that the results from serological tests are misleading due to the insensitivity of the methods used. Thus, the specific determinant on S1 may be a domain that can be represented by S1 s2 s3 s4 but due to the number and/or avidity of the antibodies to s2 s3 s4, they are not detected in the serological tests. After exposure to the second 'specific' determinant — S2 — represented as s1 S2 s3 s4 — the antibody memory cells established by the first strain are stimulated to produce antibodies to the S1 determinant. Since only a limited number of people produce antibodies to S2 in addition to S1, there must be some form of antigenic competition; earlier studies in rabbits have shown that if sufficient antigen is given a 'primary' antibody response to the second strain is induced (Fazekas and Webster, 1964).

These studies indicate that it is not possible at this time to say with certainty whether the different antigenic determinants on the hemagglutinin molecule of influenza viruses represent separate domains or whether the determinants are in a single domain. The available evidence suggests that the domain(s) are located near the hydrophilic ends of the molecule (Wrigley *et al.*, 1977), but at this time the amino acid sequences specifying the antigenic determinants are unknown.

Acknowledgements
This work was supported by Contract No. AI 42510 and Research Grant No. AI 08831 from The National Institute of Allergy and Infectious Diseases. The studies in humans were done by Drs. R. B. Couch and J. A. Kasel at Baylor College of Medicine, Houston, Texas, U.S.A.

REFERENCES
FAZEKAS DE ST. GROTH, S. (1961) Aust. J. Exp. Biol. Med. Sci. *39*, 563-582.
FAZEKAS DE ST. GROTH, S. and WEBSTER, R. G. (1966) J. Exp. Med. *124*, 347-361.
FRANCIS, T. Jr., DAVENPORT, F. M. and HENNESSY, A. V. (1953) Trans. Ass. Amer. Phycns. *66*, 231-239.
LAVER, W. G., DOWNIE, J. C. and WEBSTER, R. G. (1974) Virology *59*, 230-244.

SCHULMAN, J. L. (1975) in 'The Influenza Viruses and Influenza' (Kilbourne, E. D., ed.) pp. 373, Academic Press, New York.

SCHULZE, I. T. (1975) in 'The Influenza Viruses and Influenza' (Kilbourne, E. D., ed.) pp. 53, Academic Press, New York.

VIRELIZIER, J. L., POSTLETHWAITE, R., SCHILD, G. C. and ALLISON, A. C. (1974a) J. Exp. Med. *140*, 1559-1570.

VIRELIZIER, J. L., ALLISON, A. C. and SCHILD, G. C. (1974b) J. Exp. Med. *140*, 1571-1578.

WEBSTER, R. G. (1968) Immunology *14*, 39-52.

WRIGLEY, N. G., LAVER, W. G. and DOWNIE, J. C. (1977) J. Mol. Biol. *109*, 405-421.

THE DELINEATION OF ANTIGENIC DETERMINANTS OF THE HEMAGGLUTININ OF INFLUENZA A VIRUSES BY MEANS OF MONOCLONAL ANTIBODIES

Walter Gerhard

Summary

The antigenicity of various viral hemagglutinins (HA) of the H0 and H1 subtypes was analyzed by means of monoclonal anti-HA antibodies of BALB/c origin which were produced *in vitro*. Anti-HA(PR8) antibodies were able to discriminate 44 (groups of) determinants, one specific for the HA of PR8 and the others present (in a crossreactive form) on a variable number of HA of the heterologous influenza virus strains. It was estimated that the 9 antigenically related HA included in the analysis represent a minimum of $(2)^7$ antigenic determinants that are recognized by the BALB/c immune system, implying that the individual HA may contain approximately 15 to 65 distinct determinants.

Introduction

It has been shown previously (Gerhard, 1976) that monoclonal anti-HA (PR8) antibodies were able to delineate 14 (groups of) antigenic determinants on the HA of PR8, WSE, MEL, BEL and CAM: one specific for the HA(PR8) and 13 present on either one or several of the heterologous HA. It was postulated, however, that this estimate represented a minimum, and that by increasing the number of related viruses used in the analysis new determinants would most likely be evidenced. The number of novel determinants might, however, be expected to decrease with each additional virus employed. In order to test this point, an antigenic analysis including 4 additional viruses (BH, Hickcox, Weiss and FM1) was performed.

In the present study, 183 monoclonal anti-HA(PR8) antibodies delineated a total of 44 HA-determinants. The number of distinguishable HA-determinants, as expected, asymptotically approached an upper limit of $(2)^6$ as the number of viruses used in the analysis was increased. The results suggest that the 9 viruses included in the analysis represent a total of approximately $(2)^7$ distinct HA-determinants recognized by the BALB/c immune system.

Materials and Methods

Virus

The following influenza virus strains were used: WSE (A/WSE/33 (H0N1)), PR8 (A/PR/8/43 (H0N1)), BH (A/BH/35 (H0N1)), MEL (A/Melbourne/35 (H0N1)), Hick. (A/Hickcox/40 (H0N1)), BEL (A/Bellamy/42 (H0N1)), Weiss (A/Weiss/43 (H0N1)), CAM (A/Cam./46 (H1N1)), FM1 (A/FM/1/47 (H1N1)).

All viruses were grown in the allantoic cavity of chicken eggs and were purified as described previously (Gerhard *et al.*, 1975) before being used in the antigenic analysis.

Production of Monoclonal Antibodies

Monoclonal anti-viral antibodies were produced in the splenic fragment culture system as described previously (Gerhard, 1976; Gerhard *et al.*, 1975). Briefly, a limiting number of spleen cells from BALB/c mice previously primed with PR8 were transferred into lethally irradiated syngeneic recipient mice. Splenic fragments of the recipients were stimulated *in vitro* with PR8. Provided a sufficiently small number of PR8-primed spleen cells is transferred, each splenic focus (i.e., anti-viral antibody producing fragment) is likely to originate from a single precursor B cell which, upon antigenic stimulation, generates a clone of anti-viral antibody secreting plasma cells.

Application of Antibodies in the Antigenic Analysis

The culture fluid from each individual splenic focus, harvested in the course of its entire lifespan *in vitro*, was pooled before being analyzed in the indirect solid phase radioimmunoassay (RIA). The RIA was performed as previously described (Gerhard *et al.*, 1975) except for the use of the immunoadsorbent, which was in the form of purified virus coupled to the walls of soft plastic plates (Rosenthal *et al*, 1973). The analysis of each antibody clone was done in the following sequence: First, the anti-HA specificity of the antibody clone was determined in the RIA on the basis of its interaction with PR8(H0N1) and the hybrid virus Eq-PR8 (Heq2N1) as previously described (Gerhard, 1976). Second, the class of the anti-HA antibody was determined in the RIA. The class-specific antisera (Meloy Laboratories, Inc., Springfield, VA) were purified on the corresponding mouse-Ig-bromoacetyl-cellulose and iodinated by the chloramine-T method (Robbins *et al.*, 1967; Klinman and Aschinazi, 1974). Third, each antibody clone was tested in the RIA for its crossreaction with the various viruses. Each assay was done in quadruplicate against the homologous and in duplicate against the various heterologous viruses. The crossreaction was analyzed with iodinated class-specific antisera (label) which were directed against the predominant antibody class secreted by the given splenic focus.

A reactivity type (RT) was assigned to each monoclonal antibody on the basis of its crossreaction in the RIA (Gerhard, 1976). The RT is defined, briefly, as follows: a heterologous interaction is regarded as positive (+) if it equals or exceeds 10% and negative (-) if it is less than 10% (usually not detectable) of the homologous virus antibody interaction. Generally, these RT correlate with the ability of the heterologous viruses to cross-stimulate *in vitro* those precursor B cells that will give rise to an antibody clone which is crossreactive in the RIA with the cross-stimulating virus (W. Gerhard; manuscript in preparation).

Results

Antibody-class and Reactivity Type (RT)

If the RT of each monoclonal anti-HA antibody is a function of its energy of interaction with the homologous and the various heterologous HA (Gerhard, 1976; Gerhard *et al.*, 1975) the RT might depend to a considerable extent on the antibody-class. IgM, for example, which is a pentamer of the 4-chain Ig subunit has 10 combining sites and therefore, has the potential of making decavalent interactions as opposed to the tetravalent interaction of dimeric disulfide bonded serum IgA or the divalent interactions of IgG and monomeric IgA.

Approximately one-third of the secondary splenic foci secreted anti-HA antibodies of the IgM class. In most instances, however, IgM represented only a small fraction (⟨10%) of the total anti-HA antibodies secreted by a given focus. Table 1 shows that IgM foci seem to represent a random selection of the various RT observed with 183 foci (Table 2). Furthermore, the antibodies of focus number 24/68, which belonged to three different classes (IgM, IgG1 and IgG2), all exhibited the same RT. Thus, it seems unlikely that the antibody class contributes significantly to the diversity of the observed RT.

Relationship between the Number of RT and the Number of Viruses used in the Analysis

Monoclonal anti-HA(PR8) antibodies were tested in the RIA for their cross-reactivity with 8 heterologous viruses of the A0 (WSE, BH, Hickcox, BEL, Weiss) and A1 (CAM, FM1) sub-types. The enormous diversity of RT exhibited by these antibodies is shown in Table 2. The following analysis is based on the RT of the 144 anti-HA antibodies (Table 2) and an additional 39 anti-HA clones tested with all viruses except FM1.

The number of RT exhibited by the 183 anti-HA(PR8) antibody clones was related (Table 3) to increasing numbers of heterologous viruses included in the analysis. The sequence in which additional viruses were employed paralleled

Table 1

Splenic Focus No.	Class of Antibody	Antibody-Class and RT Reactivity Type Observed in RIA									
		PR8	WSE	BH	MEL	Hick.	BEL	Weiss	CAM	FM1	Denver
24/3	IgM	+	-	-	-	-	-	-	-	-	-
24/35	IgM	+	-	-	-	-	-	-	-	-	-
23/32	IgM	+	-	-	+	-	-	-	-	-	-
23/37	IgM	+	-	-	+	-	+	+	-	-	-
24/68	IgM	+	+	+	+	+	-	+	+	+	-
id.	IgG1	+	+	+	+	+	-	+	+	+	-
id.	IgG2	+	+	+	+	+	-	+	+	+	-

The binding of the anti-HA (PR8) antibodies to the indicated viruses in the RIA was analyzed with iodinated class-specific anti-IgM, anti-G1 or anti-G2 respectively.

Table 2

Number of Anti-HA (PR8) Antibody Clones Exhibiting Indicated RT

PR8	WSE	BH	Mel	Hick.	Bel	Weiss	Cam	FM1	RT
+	+	+	+	+	+	+	+	+	5
+	.	+	+	+	+	+	+	+	15
+	+	.	+	+	+	+	+	.	6
+	+	+	.	+	.	+	+	+	2
+	+	+	+	.	+	.	+	+	1
+	.	+	+	.	+	+	+	.	7
+	+	+	+	+	+	+	.	+	4
+	+	+	+	+	+	+	.	.	1
+	+	+	+	+	+	.	.	+	5
+	+	+	+	+	+	.	+	.	1
+	.	.	.	+	+	+	.	.	1
+	+	+	+	+	.	+	+	.	1
.	+	+	+	.	+	+	+	+	1
.	.	+	.	+	+	+	+	+	2
+	+	+	.	+	+	+	.	+	3
+	+	+	+	+	+	+	.	.	1
+	+	+	+	+	.	+	.	+	1
.	.	.	+	+	.	.	+	.	1
+	+	+	+	+	+	.	.	.	7
+	+	+	.	.	.	.	+	.	1
+	+	+	+	+	.	+	.	+	3
+	+	+	+	+	.	.	+	.	1
+	+	+	.	.	.	.	.	+	2
+	.	.	.	.	.	.	.	.	2
+	+	.	.	.	.	.	.	.	17
+	.	.	.	.	.	.	.	.	31

Table 3

Number of RT in Relation to Number of Viruses Used in Analysis

Heterologous Viruses Used in Analysis (Cumulative Number of Viruses)	Number of Clones Analyzed	Number of Reactivity Types (RT)		
		Expected		Observed
		Total*	Poisson**	
WSE + BH (2)	183	4	4	4
as above + MEL (3)	183	8	8	8
as above + Hick. (4)	183	16	16	16
as above + BEL (5)	183	32	32	25
as above + Weiss (6)	183	64	60	38
as above + CAM (7)	183	128	97	44
as above + FM1 (8)	144	256	110	44

* Total theoretically possible number of different RT equals $(2)^v$, where v is the number of heterologous viruses used in the analysis.

** Expected number of different RT is determined according to the Poisson distribution: assuming that the probability to occur is identical for each RT, the probability P of any RT not to occur $P(x=0) = \frac{\lambda^x}{x!} e^{-\lambda}$, where λ equals $\frac{\text{total number of clones analyzed}}{(2)^v}$.

Thus, the expected number of RT (Poisson) equals $(2)^v - (2)^v \times P(x=0)$.

the chronology of their isolation, starting with WSE (1933) and ending with FM1 (1947). The relationship between the number of novel RT observed and the number of viruses employed, however, was not significantly influenced by the sequence in which each virus was included in the analysis.

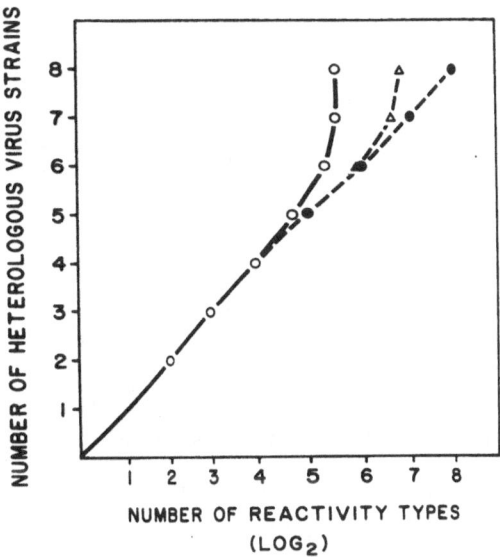

Figure 1

Relationship between the observed (O) and expected (total: ●, Poisson △) number of different cross-reactivity patterns (RT) and the number of heterologous virus strains used in the analysis.

Table 3 and Figure 1 show that the number of observed and expected RT coincide when up to 4 viruses (WSE, BH, MEL, Hickcox) are included in the analysis. Thereafter, however, fewer and fewer novel RT are observed with each additional virus. Thus, the number of observed RT seemed to asymptotically approach a limit. It is concluded that the number of observed RT would not be likely to exceed $(2)^6$ even if the analysis would be extended to more anti-HA (PR8) antibodies and additional crossreactive viruses.

Theoretical Extension of the Analysis to Include Other Anti-HA (H0 and H1) Antibodies

So far, the analysis dealt only with anti-HA (PR8) antibodies. If anti-HA antibodies raised against each of the 8 'heterologous' viruses would be analyzed for their crossreactivity they would theoretically generate no more than 255 new RT, none of which would react with the HA of PR8. By analogy to the results observed with anti-HA (PR8) antibodies, which seemed unable to exhibit more than 64 of 256 possible RT, it might thus be assumed that of the 255 possible new RT*, a maximum of approximately 64 would be exhibited by the additional anti-HA (H0 and H1) antibodies. If so, monoclonal BALB/c antibodies would be able to distinguish a total of approximately 130 determinants on the 9 HA.

Discussion

The definition of an antigenic determinant is always relative to a given population of antibody combining sites and, unless the monovalent antigen-antibody interaction can be expressed in absolute terms as free energy of binding, it depends also on the assay system used in the delineation of the determinant(s) (Crumpton, 1974). An additional degree of relativity is imposed by the possibility that individual antisera raised against a single complex protein antigen such as the hemagglutinin (HA) of influenza may vary considerably with regard to their composition (relative proportion of various antibody populations). An idea of the large variety of distinct anti-viral antibody populations has been provided by the studies of Fazekas de St. Groth (1967) and is supported here.

The recent studies of Laver *et al.* (1974) and Virelizier *et al.* (1974) have clearly demonstrated the existance of 2 groups of anti-HA antibody populations: one, reacting exclusively with the homologous HA and the other reacting with homologous and one or several heterologous HA. It was concluded that the viral HA contains at least 2 (groups of) antigenic determinants.

The above observations have been extended by means of monoclonal anti-HA antibodies which allowed the dissection of the 'common' antigenic area into many of its individual, 'partially shared' determinants.

In the present study, monoclonal anti-HA (PR8) antibodies were able to discriminate, in the form of the various types of crossreactions (RT), 43 determinants that were expressed on one or several of the heterologous HA. The above estimate is, however, a minimum for the reasons outlined in the Results section. Thus, taking into account the limited number of viruses and antibodies used in the analysis as well as the fact that only anti-HA antibodies reacting with the

Total possible number of RT if 9 viruses and anti-HA antibodies raised against each virus are included in analysis =

$$\sum_{i=1}^{g} \binom{g}{i} = 511$$

Additional RT = 511 - 256 = 255

HA of PR8 were included, the total number of determinants that could conceivably be distinguished by BALB/c anti-HA antibodies was estimated as $(2)^7$. It is difficult to deduce from this estimate the number of distinct determinants present on the HA of any given virus strain. The number of unique determinants per HA must, however, be smaller than the above estimate. Approximately $(2)^6$ determinants per HA would be expected if positive interaction of a RT with a given HA would always imply the presence of the determinant delineated by the given RT. On the other hand, assuming that different RT can interact, in some cases, with the same determinant on a given HA, the number of distinct determinants per HA could be considerably smaller. It should, however, not be less than 14-15 ($(2)^7 \div 9$).

The present estimate of 15 to 65 HA-determinants per HA-spike seems very large, especially if all determinants are localized, as suggested by the study of Wrigley *et al.* (1977), on a narrow band surrounding the HA-spike immediately below its hydrophilic tip. It should be remembered, however, that the definition of an antigenic determinant does not imply any characterization of the determinants with regard to their location or their mutual topographic relationship. Indeed, it is conceivable that these various determinants represent only the combinations of a limited number of contact points (localized in a 'small' antigenic area) with which the antibody combining sites of the various RT interact.

More important, however, than estimating the number of HA-determinants is the demonstration that the present methodology is able to dissect the complex antigenic relationship among H0 and H1 into its integral components. Thus, antigenic variation can now be monitored at the level of individual determinants which, ultimately, may lead to a better understanding of the rules that govern the mechanism of antigenic drift.

Acknowledgement

I wish to thank Mrs. Maureen Carey and Mrs. Roseann Mazzola for their help throughout this study and to Miss Linda Buettner for her help in the preparation of this manuscript.

REFERENCES

CRUMPTON, M. J. (1974) in 'The Antigens' (Ed., Sela, M.) Vol. II, 1-78. Academic Press.

FAZEKAS DE ST. GROTH, S. (1967) Cold Spring Harbor Symposia on Quantative Biology, Vol. 32, 525-536.

GERHARD, W. (1976) J. Exp. Med. *144*, 985-995.

GERHARD, W., BRACIALE, T. J. and KLINMAN, N. R. (1975) Eur. J. Immunol. *5*, 720.

KLINMAN, N. R. and ASCHINAZI, G. (1971) J. Immunol. *106*, 1338-1344.

LAVER, W. G., DOWNIE, J. C. and WEBSTER, R. G. (1974) Virology *59*, 230-244.

ROBBINS, J. B., HAIMOVICH, J. and SELA, M. (1967) Immunochemistry *4*, 11-22.

ROSENTHAL, I. D., HAYASHI, K. and NOTKINS, A. L. (1973) Appl. Microbiol. *25*, 567-573.

VIRELIZIER, J. L., ALLISON, A. C. and SCHILD, G. C. (1974) J. exp. Med. *140*, 1571-1578.

WRIGLEY, N. G., LAVER, W. G. and DOWNIE, J. C. (1977) J. Mol. Biol. *109*, 405-421.

ANTIGENIC, ADAPTIVE AND ADSORPTIVE VARIANTS OF THE INFLUENZA A HEMAGGLUTININ

S. Fazekas de St. Groth

The material I wish to present falls in two parts. First, an analysis of mutants obtained by various selection procedures in the laboratory and, second, comparison of these findings with what happens in Nature, by intention at least, a synthesis.

I   Laboratory Mutants

Selection under Pressure of Antibody

A proper method for defining the scope and frequency of mutations must separate the mutants from the parental input, must isolate them singly and must operate under known, specified selective pressure.

These requirements are met by using a large number (usually 640 per experiment) of small host tissue units (about 10^6 cells of either the surviving allantois or of primary calf kidney cultures) and distributing over them a mixture of 10^{10}-10^{11} ID_{50} of virus and the most avid fraction of hyperimmune antibody. The concentration of antibody is so adjusted that the virus is overneutralized by a factor of 10 to 1000. Under these conditions reisolation of parental virus has a probability of less than 1 in 100, and the chance of two isolates coinciding in the same tissue unit is also well below 1 in 100. The system is incubated in a synthetic medium, in the absence of serum, for 68 hr at $35^{\circ}C$. At the end of this period a drop of 5% sterile fowl red cells is added to each cup, and the contents of those showing agglutination are isolated. The isolates are cloned both in the presence and absence of the selecting serum, and grown to titer in the same host system.

The growth characteristics of these isolates were tested in single-cycle experiments and they were classified antigenically by the use of a battery of hyperimmune sera. All sera, including those used at the selection stage, were made against immunogens that shared no host component. Thus for selection tests in allantoic cells, rabbits were immunized with purified whole virus or its isolated hemagglutinin derived from calf kidney cultures, while antisera to egg-grown immunogens were used for selection in calf kidney cultures. Since antisera are heterogenous, being made up of a large variety of antibodies more or less complementary to the stimulating antigen, they are bound to contain subsets capable of reacting with any emerging mutant. Thus, while these mutants may stand a better chance of escaping neutralization than the parent, their survival is by no means certain. Discrimination can be greatly improved by selecting under the most avid fraction of the antibody population. To this end the sera were chromatographed on an affinity column containing the homologous antigen (Fazekas de St. Groth, 1967), and the fraction eluted between pH 2.65 and 2.25 used for neutralization. This fraction, usually 1.4 - 4% of the specific antibody globulins, had an equilibrium constant of 10^{11} molecules/ml or better, with no sign of inhomogeneity, i.e., with the equilibrium constant independent of serum concentration.

Adsorptive Mutants

The majority of isolates surviving under low selective pressure turned out to be antigenically indistinguishable from their parent. The commonly used tests (neutralization or inhibition of hemagglutination) can be very misleading in this respect. These mutants bind more firmly to neuraminyl glycoproteins and thus in a ternary competition the equilibrium will be shifted in favour of the host or indicator cell. The difference disappears in binary tests, such as fixation of complement with the V-antigen or passive agglutination of virus-coated erythrocytes. Antigenic identity follows also from results of cross absorption tests: they show complete reciprocity in all combinations.

The nature of mutation is revealed by placing the isolates in the receptor gradient (Archetti and Horsfall, 1950). Adsorptive mutants take up a position below the parent, i.e., erythrocytes treated with neuraminidase or metaperiodate to a level where they are not agglutinated anymore by the parental virus, are still agglutinated by the mutant.

Adsorptive mutants have usually the same growth characteristics as their parent. When we found any difference, it was always a higher cyclic yield by the mutant.

The frequency of such mutations is at least 10^{-8}, but an exact rate cannot be defined since – and this is a basic characteristic of adsorptive mutants – the success of isolation is inversely proportional to the antibody concentration. Thus if a preparation of, say 10^9 ID_{50} is overneutralized by a factor of 3 or 5, about 10 adsorptive mutants can be isolated; the same dose of virus overneutralized by a factor of 10-20 will yield none, even in repeated trials.

Table 1

PROPERTIES OF ADSORPTIVE MUTANTS

1. Cross reactions of sera

	in ternary tests		binary tests	
Antigen	anti-parent	anti-mutant	anti-parent	anti-mutant
Parent	= 100	120 - 250	= 100	100 ± 10
Mutant	30 - 75	= 100	100 ± 10	= 100

2. Cross reactions of sera absorbed with

	parent		mutant	
Antigen	anti-parent	anti-mutant	anti-parent	anti-mutant
Parent	-	-	-	-
Mutant	-	-	-	-

- = less than 2%

3. Cross reactions with other subtypes: same as parents

4. Position in receptor gradient: significantly lower than parent

5. Growth characteristics: same or faster than parent
Cyclic yield: 200-300/cell
Median cycle time: 8.5 hours

6. Frequency of isolation: between 10^{-8} and 10^{-11}, depends on the selecting serum concentration

7. Sequential selection: successful

The locus of adsorptive mutations is not within the epitope (the area of an antigen with which the complementary region of an antibody molecule, the paratope, makes direct contact). This we know from equilibrium measurements where the same number of antibody molecules and the same equilibrium constant is estimated by the parental and mutant antigen and, more compellingly, from thermodynamic measurements where the two antigens are indistinguishable by changes in latent heat and entropy when tested against any particular serum. It follows that the epitope through which neutralization takes place is either completely distinct from the area through which virus and cell are bound, or it is a subset of the adsorptive area. This question can be decided only by performing similar measurements on antigenic mutants, but in the meantime we may note that independent adsorptive mutants are frequently isolated under pressure of antibody, and it is well to keep this fact in mind when trying to piece together the natural history of these viruses.

Hierarchic Mutants

The first class of true antigenic mutants arises with a frequency of $1.5 - 3 \times 10^{-9}$ and this rate is independent of the concentration of the selecting serum. In fact, the standard selection test is set up at four dilutions of serum and we take it as presumptive evidence for having eliminated both parental virus and adsorptive mutants if the number of isolates is roughly the same at each level of overneutralization.

That these isolates differ antigenically from their parent is evident from their cross reactions, both in ternary and binary tests. The relationship is peculiar: sera raised against a mutant neutralize the parent almost as well as do anti-parental sera, while anti-parental sera are strikingly less efficient against their mutants. Such asymmetric cross reactions define a hierarchic order — hence the name of these mutants — with the offspring antigenically outranking the parent, being senior to it.

This junior-senior pattern holds for each of the hundreds of antigenic mutants we have isolated from two subtypes. It is best interpreted by assuming a substitution within the epitope such that a bulkier amino acid in the mutant offers steric hindrance to antibodies directed against the parental epitope. On this model a smaller fraction of anti-junior antibodies should be capable of reacting with senior antigens than the other way round; hence the asymmetry of crossing. It is also implied that junior antigens should bind almost all classes of anti-junior sera. This phenomenon has been widely noted for field strains standing in junior-senior relation (Archetti and Horsfall, 1950; Fazekas de St. Groth,1967,1969a, 1969b, 1970; Friedewald, 1944; Hilleman, 1951; Isaacs and Andrewes, 1951; Takátsy and Fürész, 1956; Taylor, 1949); our absorption tests show that it holds equally for hierarchic mutants.

What is more difficult to interpret is that most pairs of antigenic mutants derived from the same parent give such lopsided cross reactions with each other, too. This would imply that substitutions are occurring preferentially or exclusiv-

Table 2

PROPERTIES OF HIERARCHIC MUTANTS

1. Cross reactions of sera in

Antigen	ternary tests		binary tests	
	anti-parent	anti-mutant	anti-parent	anti-mutant
Parent	= 100	75 - 100	= 100	75 - 100
Mutant	20 - 50	= 100	20 - 50	= 100

2. Cross reactions of sera absorbed with

Antigen	parent		mutant	
	anti-parent	anti-mutant	anti-parent	anti-mutant
Parent	-	-	50 - 75	-
Mutant	-	3 - 15	-	-

- = less than 2%

3. Cross reactions with other subtypes: distant, same as parent

4. Position in receptor gradient: same as parent $\pm$ 10%

5. Growth characteristics: usually slower than parent
Cyclic yield: 50-200/cell
Median cycle time: 9-15 hours

6. Frequency of isolation: $1.5 - 3 \times 10^{-9}$, independent of selective pressure

7. Sequential selection: Successful over 2-4 generations

ely at the same locus within the epitope, thus running counter to the normal assumption of randomness. Survivors of random substitutions may well score as senior to the parent, but they should display no hierarchic distinctions among themselves. This, however, is not what we find.

Most hierarchic mutants take up positions in the receptor gradient close to their parent; if there is any measurable difference, it may lie in either direction. This suggests that the antigenic determinant plays only a minor role in defining the adsorptive behavior of a particular strain. But, since there are adsorptive shifts correlated with antigenic change, it also suggests that the epitope forms part of the larger adsorptive area.

Hierarchic mutants do not as a rule grow as well as their parent; their cycle time is usually longer and the cyclic yield reduced, often markedly. They differ in this respect from adsorptive mutants which thrive in the tissue of isolation; whereas antigenic mutants tend to score as deadapted.

Bridging Mutants

The second class of antigenic mutants is much rarer than the hierarchic kind. They are isolated with a frequency between 10^{-11} and 10^{-12}, but this is no more than a minimum estimate since, due to their growth characteristics, some members of this group might not reach hemagglutinating levels in the selective passage and thus escape detection. The rate of isolation is independent of the degree of overneutralization by antibody fully complementary to the parent. Unfractionated sera, however, often contain quite firmly binding antibodies that will neutralize these mutants; when such are used for selection, the success of isolating bridging mutants becomes serum-dependent.

Cross reactions between parent and mutant, in both binary and ternary tests, establish clear junior-senior relations. The number of bridging mutants we have isolated is too small to allow general conclusions, but the heterologous titers were rather lower than found with hierarchic mutants. This impression is strengthened by cross absorption tests where both parent and mutant are less efficient in binding the heterologous antibody.

When comparing bridging mutants among themselves or bridging and hierarchic mutants derived from the same parent, the most common pattern is a distant (⟨20%) and symmetric cross reactivity. Some of the bridging mutants react also outside their subtype, a result never found with the many hierarchic mutants we tested. Both of these features point to substitutions at different loci within the epitope. They renew the question why such apparently random substitutions are recovered with frequencies about a hundred times lower than hierarchic substitutions which, restricted to one locus, should be less probable.

Bridging mutants do not grow well. Compared to the parent, their median cycle time is at least twice as long and their cyclic yield often less than a tenth. This holds for all bridging strains we have recovered to date and, even to produce enough virus for a more detailed study of its properties, each of them had to be readapted to the selfsame tissue in which it was isolated.

Table 3

PROPERTIES OF BRIDGING MUTANTS

1. Cross reactions of sera

Antigen	ternary tests in		binary tests	
	anti-parent	anti-mutant	anti-parent	anti-mutant
Parent	= 100	40 - 75	= 100	40 - 75
Mutant	10 - 30	= 100	10 - 30	= 100

2. Cross reactions of sera absorbed with

Antigen	parent		mutant	
	anti-parent	anti-mutant	anti-parent	anti-mutant
Parent	-	-	60 - 90	-
Mutant	-	30 - 50	-	-

    - = less than 2%

3. Cross reactions with other subtypes: frequent broader than parent

4. Position in receptor gradient: same as parent $\pm$ 10%

5. Growth characteristics: much slower than parent
Cyclic yield: $\langle 5-25/$cell
Median cycle time: 12 - 24 hours

6. Frequency of isolation: $\langle 10^{-11}$, independent of selective pressure

7. Sequential selection: usually unsuccessful

Sequential Selection

By using the most avid fraction of antisera prepared mutants, selection can be carried through further rounds. We have done that, starting with the most junior members of two subtypes, and from the large body of data (Fazekas de St. Groth, 1970; Fazekas de St. Groth and Hannoun, 1973; Fazekas de St. Groth, 1975; Fazekas de St. Groth and Tees, 1975) some general conclusions may be drawn.

1. The frequency of adsorptive mutants is roughly the same at any level and occasionally even more firmly binding forms (presumably double mutants) can be selected from first-generation adsorptive mutants. Such mutations are readily recognized by the difference of cross reactions in binary and ternary tests, by the complete and reciprocal absorption of antiparental and antimutant sera, and by their shift in the receptor gradient.

2. Sequential antigenic mutants stand in hierarchic relation to their whole lineage: they score as senior not only to the immediate but to all their predecessors, and junior to all their descendants.

3. Comparisons outside the direct line of descent show no consistent hierarchic order. Indeed, indistinguishable antigenic patterns may turn up in different branches of the family and may be reached in a different number of steps or through different intermediates.

4. After two to four steps of sequential selection the series comes to an end: the same technique which selected mutants with a frequency of the order 10^{-9} abruptly drops to a rate of less than 10^{-12}. The terminal mutant still belongs to the same subtype as the original parent.

5. While there are several different epitopes distinguishable among first- and second-generation antigenic mutants, they tend to give rise to the same terminal forms.

6. Bridging mutants, even though only one step removed from the most junior member of the antigenic hierarchy, generally behave as terminal forms. The single exception we found could be carried only one step further before stopping to yield under the pressure of antibody.

7. No bridging mutants could be isolated from any of the second-, third- or fourth-generation of hierarchic mutants we have tested.

Antigenic mutants thus appear to form an ordered, degenerate, convergent and bounded set which is independent of the set of adsorptive mutants. The observations have been interpreted in terms of substitutions within a hydrophobic area (Fazekas de St. Groth, 1975), a hypothesis supported by the fact that the influenza A virus-antibody combination is entirely entropy-driven (Fazekas de St. Groth, 1962; Fazekas de St. Groth and Gerhard, in preparation), i.e., exacts hydrophobic interactions between epitope and paratope.

Selection under Environmental Pressure: Adaptive Mutants

Basically all laboratory strains of influenza are adaptive mutants of epidemic strains since, as has been convincingly shown some thirty years ago (Burnet and Bull, 1943), growth in the allatois amounts to selection of mutants, usually sequential selection. In fact, the starting member of our series from the present subtype, NT 60/1968, is demonstrably different from the antigenically identical HK 1/1968 strain: it has a shorter cycle time while its cyclic yield is about twelve times higher. As we have seen, hierarchic mutants tend to grow more slowly than their parent, this disadvantage becoming increasingly evident in the more senior forms. Bridging mutants are even less well adapted, most of them just managing a positive rate of growth.

For the study of adaptive mutations we used the technique of skim passage (Fazekas de St. Groth and Tees, 1975). The principle is based on the correlation between long cycle times and low cyclic yields. What we do then is to infect a tissue with a high dose of virus and skim off the yield at a time when about 50% of an adapted virus would be released but much less than 1% of an unadapted one. By repeating the process a few times we invariably get better-growing strains, as well as a rough idea of the number of mutational steps required and the frequency of such mutants.

1. The original parental strain, NT60, did not grow well in calf kidney cultures. We did four adaptive experiments, and in each it took two separate mutational events to reduce the cycle time. The frequency of mutants was 10^{-7} or better at each stage. The adapted forms, however, were not identical: one had a cyclic yield of 250, the other three lay between 80 and 150. This property was stable on standard passaging and the low yielders could not be improved by further rounds of skim passage.

2. Hierarchic mutants isolated in the allantois could be usually readapted in a single step, at an imput of ca. 10^7 ID_{50}. A minority, and that largely restricted to senior forms, needed two steps, while one terminal mutant could not be successfully readapted. To our surprise, most of the original isolates grew as well in calf kidney cultures as did their parent, i.e., the

antigenic change was correlated with deadaptation from one host tissue (actually, the one in which they were isolated), while they remained adapted to a second host tissue.

3.   Many hierarchic mutants reverted to the parental or even more junior antigenic type if the adaptive passage was run in the absence of antibody against the parent. This finding is paradoxical since with a forward mutational rate of about 10^{-9} the frequency of back-mutations would be expected to be of the same order, and thus adaptive changes should be found a hundred times more frequently than antigenic reversions.

4.   The majority of bridging strains required at least two, mostly three skim passages before mutants with cycle times approaching the parental could be isolated. Even these forms were only partly adapted as their cycle yield often still remained well below the parent's and could not be improved by further skim passages.

While adsorptive and antigenic mutations can be formally assigned to the HA molecule – the isolated hemagglutinin gives the same distinguishing reactions as the whole virus particle – the placing of adaptive mutations is more difficult. The argument in favour of the HA molecule rests on the correlation of antigenic change with often severe deadaptation. On this hypothesis adaptation would amount to one or more suppressor mutations, i.e. the functional conformation of the molecule (which has been distorted by the antigenic change) would be reestablished by compensating substitutions outside the antigenic area. This concept is argued against by the experience of co-passaging adapted and unadapted strains and isolating a well-growing 'recombinant' which carries the HA of the unadapted partner. The locus of this particular kind of adaptive mutation might be pinpointed by finding out more about the chemical structure of the HA molecule, but the more general issue of adaptation may involve several viral products and their interactions.

II   Field Strains

The epidemiology of influenza A is still far from fully understood. We know, since the mid-thirties, that the virus is variable and, since the mid-fourties, that some of the changes are so abrupt as to define antigenic subtypes. There are consistent differences even within subtypes, as recognised more recently (Dowdle et al., 1974): the first few pandemics are homogenous (i.e., caused by the same or very similar viruses the world over), while the second phase is inhomogeneous, with several distinguishable strains responsible for often simultaneous local outbreaks. Retrospective serology puts limits on this variability, suggesting both that the number of subtypes is limited and that they are linked in a secular cycle of about 70 years (Davenport *et al.*, 1953, 1967, 1969; Davenport and Hennessy, 1958; Francis, 1952, 1960; Fukumi, 1969, 1970; Marine and Workman, 1969; Marine *et al.*, 1969; Masurel, 1967, 1968, 1969a, 1969b; Masurel and Mulder, 1966; Mulder and Masurel, 1958; Zakstelskaja *et al.*, 1969).

Each of these features is, to say the least, unusual for a pathogen in equilibrium with its environment. What remains to be done, then, is to see whether events in the field can be interpreted in terms of what we have learnt by isolating mutants in the laboratory.

The Hierarchic Phase of a Subtype

Table 4 shows the cross reactions of representative epidemic strains current in the Western hemisphere between 1968 and 1973. The pattern is asymmetric, with the high values above the main diagonal and the low ones below it. Clearly, the historic sequence defines also a hierarchic order, hence the name of this initial phase of the subtype era.

Table 4

CROSS REACTIONS OF INFLUENZA A VIRUSES

1.   Hierarchic phase of subtype A3

| | Antisera against | | | | | |
Viruses	NT 60	ENG 845	LAS	ENG 42	PRI	30c
NT 60/68	100	93	104	111	115	97
ENG 845/69	50	100	93	97	127	93
LAS/71	41	37	100	90	107	90
ENG 42/72	31	47	38	100	93	93
PRI/73	26	28	35	39	100	81
30c*	15	16	23	28	38	100

The titers are normalized to the homologous reaction (=100%), and represent means of 8-12 antisera per antigen.
* 30c, the senior laboratory mutant is included for the purposes of comparison

It should be added that the pattern would be less clear-cut if only single sera had been used in the cross reactions or if all field isolates were included. The vagaries of individual immune responses can be balanced by increasing the number of test sera, while the kinship of field strains is better understood by relating them to laboratory mutants.

The 131 mutants derived directly from the pandemic strain of 1968 could be sorted into six groups. The first two of these, making up more than half of the isolates, are adsorptive mutants and are represented in Table 5 by the strains 350/6 and 350/12. The latter is indistinguishable from the Japanese field strain AICHI, from which the 1968 vaccines were made. AICHI itself takes up a position below HK1 in the receptor gradient and is 'inhibitor resistant', another mark of changed adsorptive behavior.

The four groups of antigenic mutants are all hierarchic; 375/14 and 400/11 are very similar and junior both to 375/17 (which matches the predominant epidemic strain of the next year ENG845/69) and to 375/20 (which matches the minority field strain of 1969 ENG878). In all, the laboratory mutants covered not only the adsorptive variant of the pandemic strain and strains of the next epidemic wave, but contained also mutants which either did not occur in Nature or were missed by the conventional crude techniques of classification.

This holds also for the next generation of laboratory mutants which contained several antigenic patterns not recovered in the field. The two main epidemic strains spreading over the Western hemisphere in 1971 were matched by isolates 34c and 63c, the former a hierarchic mutant of the minority field strain of 1969 and the latter the adsorptive variant of the majority strains of 1969. The Far Eastern strains of 1971, represented by HK107, were matched by hierarchic mutants derived from either of the two groups of adsorptive mutants of the previous generation. This suggests the lineage HK1 → AICHI → HK107, and at the same time displays the degeneracy of the mutant set. Degeneracy is also evident in the appearance of equivalents of both the 1969 strains by different routes and through different intermediates. The family tree of field strains branches at ENG845/69, one limb accounting for the main epidemic strain of 1971 through ENG878/69, and the other for the rest of the 1971 strains as well as for the main field strains of the next two years.

Some terminal forms turned up already in the third generation, but these were not tested extensively. Members of the fourth generation yielded no further antigenic mutants by the standard technique of selection.

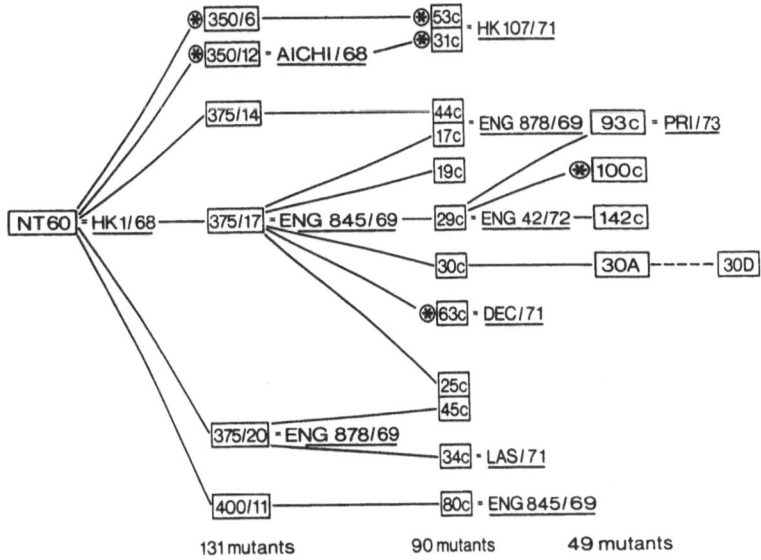

131 mutants   90 mutants   49 mutants

Figure 1

Family tree of laboratory mutants derived from A/NT 60/68 (H3N2) virus. Matching field strains are equated with the corresponding mutant. ⊛ = adsorptive mutants

The Bridging Phase of a Subtype

Even though Table 5 covers only a minor portion of distinguishable strains isolated since 1973, their cross reactions are sufficient to document the difference between the first and second half of a subtype era. Compared to the initial member of the hierarchic phase, they all score as senior; this establishes them as members of the subtype. Compared to the most senior hierarchic mutant, 30c, they all give distant and essentially symmetric cross reactions; this suggests substitutions at two loci within the antigenic area. That the second mutant locus is not the same for each of these strains follows from the results of pairwise comparisons: most cross reactions are fairly distant and more or less evenly balanced. As a consequence, the historical sequence does not impose order on this set. These epidemic strains do not continue the hierarchic series but seem to arise independently and bear marked resemblance to the bridging mutants isolated in the laboratory.

The first field strains of this group have been isolated towards the end of 1973 in New Zealand and Australia, and caused local outbreaks over the Northern winter of 1973-74. We have no laboratory mutants matching these strains and

Table 5

CROSS REACTIONS OF INFLUENZA A VIRUSES

2. Bridging phase of subtype A3

Viruses	Antisera against										
	NT 60	30c	PCH	SCOT	HAN	FIN	PR 2	ART	VIC 3	NG	VIC 112
NT 60/68*	100	97	123	76	62	68	46	57	55	62	41
30c*	15	100	19	12	15	13	24	19	24	16	18
PCH/73	12	23	100	23	22	19	26	52	18	14	22
SCOT/74	23	47	93	100	54	55	47	78	52	57	16
HAN/74	7	19	23	15	100	97	38	54	12	9	31
FIN/74	8	20	22	18	100	100	41	55	13	11	27
PR 2/74	13	25	27	24	35	30	100	35	20	18	28
ART/74	6	13	23	13	5	6	28	100	11	9	13
VIC 3/75	7	12	19	9	9	10	20	12	100	13	30
NG 75	9	15	26	13	13	12	23	19	14	100	21
VIC 112/76	7	18	24	25	10	9	19	38	35	19	100

Titers are normalized to the homologous reaction (=100%), and represent means of 4-6 sera per antigen.
* The junior and senior member of the hierarchic phase, included for comparison

the prototype, Port Chalmers/73, proved quite exceptional among influenza A viruses: it must carry a positively charged or highly bipolar group within or very close to its epitope since the combination between this virus and its antibody is characterized by -7 kcal/mole of standard enthalpy change. As a result it scores as antigenic and adsorptive mutant at the same time. The field strain behaves as a terminal form, as has been extensively tested in two laboratories (Fazekas de St. Groth and Tees, unpublished observations; Hannoun, personal communication). We succeeded however in isolating a back-mutant from it, and when that was placed under special pressure (antibody against the most senior member of the hierarchic series, covering all mutations at the subtype-locus but allowing survival of forms substituted at any other locus within the epitope), it yielded a number of bridging mutants. One of these matched the group of field strains isolated in Northern Europe (HAN/74 and FIN/74), while another proved very similar but senior to the Caribbean epidemic strain PR2/74. There is no exact equivalent among our mutants to the predominant field strain of 1975, VIC3, but the new Australian strain of 1976, VIC112, is matched by the bridging mutant D13.

The correspondence between laboratory isolates and epidemic strains of the bridging phase is thus incomplete: both sets have members not matched by the other. Yet, it seems reasonable to equate the two groups since their basic characteristics are the same and the lack of complete overlap can be accounted for by the great variety of epidemic strains on the one hand and, on the other, by the low frequency and poor growth of the laboratory isolates.

Transition between Subtypes

Each of the four new subtypes from which viruses have been isolated started with a major pandemic (1933, 1946, 1957 and 1968). By analogy, therefore, we consider the pandemics of 1889, 1900, 1910 and 1918 equally as starting points of new subtypes. The origin of the virus causing these pandemics is unknown, but we know that each of them spread in a virtually virgin population with no specific herd immunity. The transition between subtypes is abrupt: strains belonging to previous subtypes are not recovered in the field once a new subtype has taken over. Yet, there is solid evidence (Davenport *et al.*, 1969; Fukumi, 1969, 1970; Marine *et al.*, 1969; Masurel, 1969b; Zakstelskaja *et al.*, 1969) that viruses similar to subtype A2 were current between 1889 and 1900, followed over the next decade by viruses similar to subtype A3. Such circular evolution, utterly alien to Darwinian thought, implies that there are only six subtypes within influenza A, and that the next one will be similar to strains current between 1910 and 1918.

As we have no better hypothesis, the only rational approach is to look for a virus of this kind. In practicle terms this means finding a virus with which people born before 1918 are immunologically acquainted, but not those born after 1918. Since some of our bridging mutants seem to belong to no known subtype, we hoped that at least one of them would qualify by this criterion as member of the unknown subtype current between 1910 and 1918.

We did these tests on sera collected before the 1968 pandemic. This precaution was necessary since our mutants were all derived from strains of the present subtype and we had to guard against misleading cross reactions. The controls were as expected: over 90% of all sera gave positive tests with SING/57 (the most junior member of the subtype current at the time the sera were collected) while only cohorts born before 1908 reacted with NT60/68. The main finding was a group among our test antigens which reacted with over half the sera from cohorts born before 1918. This would have been a highly satisfactory result, except that the same mutants reacted also with 5-15% sera from donors born during the reign of later subtypes. It became mandatory therefore to decide whether we were dealing with some freak cross reaction, or whether there was something wrong with our basic dogma that subtypes displace each other and do not overlap.

The Age Distribution of Human Antibodies

In principle, the experiment was to tell whether a group of people born within a subtype era did or did not have antibodies against previous subtypes. The practicle test was done on sera of blood donors from Sydney's three universities. Each of the 2246 coded sera was tested against PR8/34, CAM/46, SING/57 and NT60/68 (the junior members of the four known subtypes) and against SW/31 (the putative equivalent of the 1918-19 pandemic strain). After decoding and eliminating all donors with a history of vaccination against influenza, all sera reacting outside their subtype were absorbed with each antigen and both the unbound and eluted antibody fractions titrated against each antigen.

The incidence of positive reactions is shown in Figure 2. Two things should be noted about this and the following graphs. First, that the donors born before 1946 (i.e., covering the first two subtypes) make up only 9% of the total population, while the remaining 91% was born within the era of A1 and A2 sub-types. This suggests a poor staff-to-student ratio or an increasing aversion of senior academics to be bled, or both. In practice it means that the left hand halves of the curves are less reliable than the right hand halves. And second, that some sera gave flat endpoints. Such patterns are usual for antibodies of very low avidity. These equivocal reactors are marked by the stippled areas; they were encountered, with a negligible number of exceptions, only outside the historical period of a particular subtype.

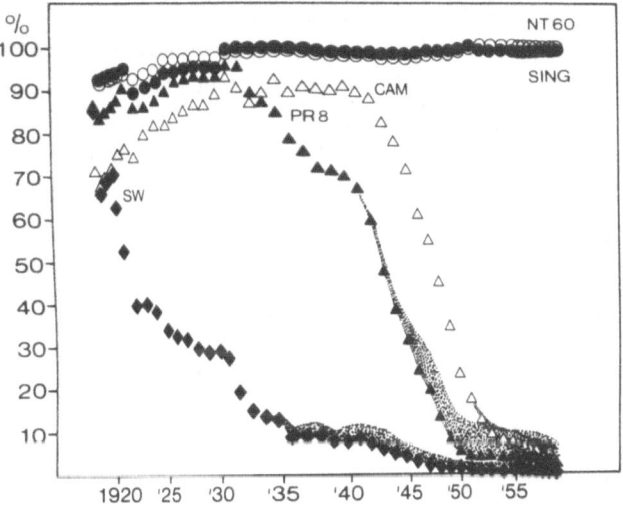

Figure 2

Moving average incidence of antibodies against the five subtypes of influenza A among 2246 healthy blood donors in 1976 (year of birth on the abscissa).

Close to 100% of the sera contained antibodies against the two recent subtypes and there is a clear temporal distribution in the incidence of reactors to previous subtypes. However, the curves for SW, PR8 and CAM do not reach the abscissa: there remain 2-5% unequivocal and up to 10% equivocal reactors among the cohorts born in the era of later subtypes.

On reexamining the evidence on which the assumption of sharp distinction between subtypes was based (Devenport *et al.*, 1953, 1967, 1969; Devenport and Hennessy, 1958; Fukumi, 1969; Marine and Workman, 1969; Marine *et al.*, 1969; Masurel, 1967, 1968, 1969a, 1969b; Masurel and Mulder, 1966; Mulder and Masurel, 1958; Zakstelskaja *et al.*, 1969), it is striking that each set of data shows the same phenomenon, with a small number of positive tests appearing where they should not be. The clearest confirmation comes from the extensive survey of reactors to SW virus, conducted under the aegis of WHO in 1976. The summary report (World Health Organization, 1977) states that 'antibodies were present at titers ⟩20 in nearly all subjects aged 50 years or more', while 'in the USA those aged 25-51 years had antibodies in only 9% and those below the age of 25 years had less than 1%'. The incidence of aberrant positives showed great regional variation: '...in Greece and Uganda no antibodies ...were detected in the age group below 30 years, while in Austria, France and Turkey no anti-bodies were detected in ages below 40 years. At the other extreme, 23% of persons aged between 30-40 years in Iceland and over 50% of those examined in Greece had antibodies'. Our experience fits perfectly within these limits and extends the observations to two more subtypes. It is remarkable that all of us, authors as well as readers, have missed or ignored a phenomenon of potentially great epidemiological significance and increasingly well documented over the past 20 years.

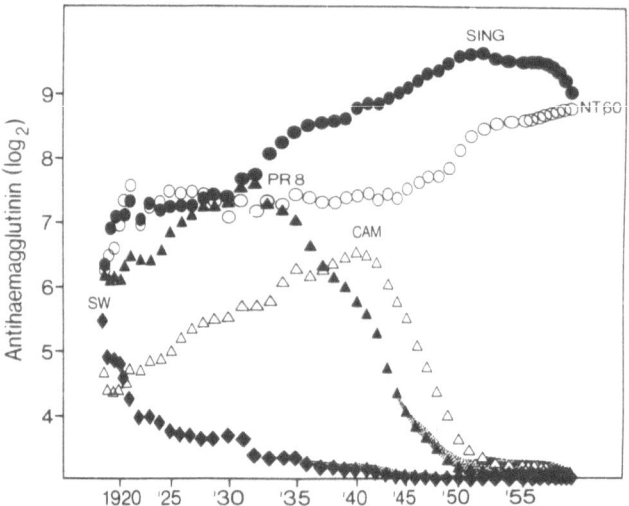

Figure 3

Average antibody titers against the five subtypes of influenza A among 2246 healthy blood donors in 1976 (year of birth on the abscissa).

When mean antibody titers rather than the incidence of positive reactions are plotted, we get a similar picture but with one additional point of information. The curves have a maximum 3-5 years before the initiating pandemic of a particular subtype. This confirms that the very young are shielded from influenza (Davenport *et al.*, 1969) and also means that the best responders, or at least those maintaining high antibody levels for the longest time, are the cohorts of the immediate pre-school age. Once again, the curves extend beyond the subtype periods and level off at 6-15% of the maximal titers.

The Nature of Illegitimate Antibodies

A rough idea about the kind of antibodies found outside the subtype era can be gained by replotting the data of Figure 3, this time averaging the positive titers only.

The positive antibody titers against each of the test strains go through a maximum immediately before or at the beginning of the respective subtype period (Figure 4). We may conclude therefore not only that the best responders are the cohorts which met that virus at an age of five years or less, but also that this differential pattern is then maintained, presumably, for life ()45 years for PR8,)37 years for CAM,)17 years for SING and by extrapolation)50 years for SW).

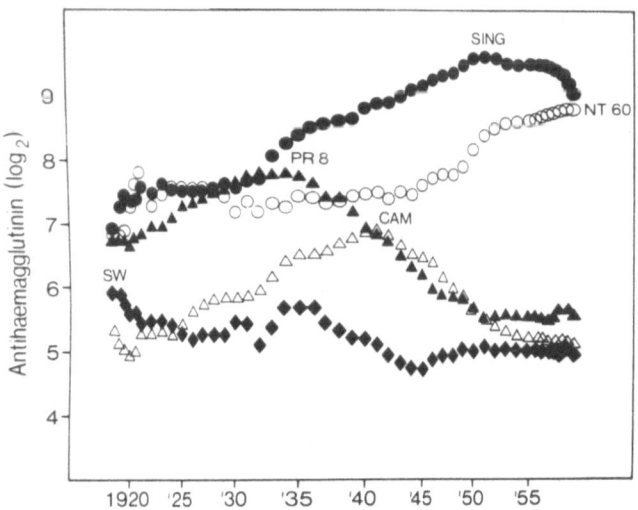

Figure 4

Average positive antibody titers against the five subtypes of influenza A among 2246 healthy blood donors in 1976 (year of birth on the abscissa). Antihemagglutinin titers of)16 are taken as positive.

What is more interesting in the present context, however, is the lack of difference between the levels at which intra- and extra-subtypic antibodies are maintained. Positive reactors outside the subtype era are fewer, but those carrying antibodies to a particular strain cannot be dated simply by their antihemagglutinin titers.

The reactions of cross-absorbed sera are more informative. Details of these tests will be published in full (Fazekas de St. Groth and Underwood, 1977); here the extra-subtypic responses to PR8 virus will be used to illustrate the general behavior of illegitimate antibodies. We fully tested 43 of these sera and compared them with a control group made up of 16 sera from cohorts 1933-45 (born within the subtype era of PR8) and 9 sera of the cohorts 1924-32 (representing the previous subtype). The dose of absorbing viruses was adjusted to $10^{14.5}$ epitopes/ml, i.e., even antibodies a hundred times less avid than the average homologous antibody would have been 90% bound, leaving only distant cross reactors in the supernate.

Absorption with the homologous virus distinguishes between legitimate and illegitimate antibodies: 21/25 of the control sera were completely absorbed by PR8 virus and the remaining 4 had on the average 5.8% antibody left in the supernate (range 2-9%). None of the sera of donors born after 1945 fell into this group. On the average about half of their antibodies remained in the supernate under conditions of our test. The quality of these supernates further differentiates among the anti-PR8 antibodies: 15 of them gave sharp endpoints (average unbound antibody 52%, range 14-81%), while the remaining 28 (containing on the average 59% antibody, range 12-93%) gave flat endpoints, indicating antibody of very low complementarity. Eluting the bound fraction, we recovered on the average 42% of the input (range 18-71%), representing the more firmly-binding antibodies of the latter group.

Adsorption with PR8 did not affect titers against the last two subtypes: only one of the 43 eluates contained some anti-SING antibody (1% of the input) and anti-NT60 was found in another eluate, at the level of 0.5%. None of the eluates of the control group gave titers against SING, while three had minimal quantities of anti-NT60 (2, 2 and 6% resp., of the input).

Twelve of the control sera had anti-CAM antibodies and six of these were partly bound also by PR8 virus (range 10-47%). Among the illegitimate anti-PR8 sera 18 had titers against CAM, but only 2 of them contained antibodies cross-reactive with PR8 (18 and 47%, resp.).

Table 6

ABSORPTION OF HUMAN SERA WITH PR 8/34 VIRUS

	Number of sera	per cent residual antibody							mean
		<1	1-10	11-30	31-50	51-70	71-90	>90	
'Legitimate antibody' Cohorts 1924-45	25	21	4	0	0	0	0	0	0.9%
'Illegitimate antibody' Cohorts 1945-59	15	0	0	1	7	3	4	0	52.5%
	28*	0	0	1	8	9	9	1	59.1%

Absorbing dose: 65 μg purified PR8 virus/ml (= 4000 HA units/ml)

* = residual antibody of very low avidity

Each of the four control sera reacting with SW proved to be partly cross-absorbable with PR8 (range 10-33%). In the extra-subtypic group 5/43 reacted with SW but of these only 3 contained cross-reactive antibody (9, 25 and 31%, resp.).

These results, and similar ones obtained with the extra-subtypic anti-SW and anti-CAM sera, allow the following conclusions:

1. A small fraction of the test sample and, according to other surveys, of the general population carries antibodies against influenza A viruses not supposed to have been current during their lifetime.

2. The portion of such extra-subtypic reactors shows great regional variation (World Health Organization, 1977). In the Australian test sample the probability of acquiring, within the first twenty years of life, antibodies against one of the three preceding subtypes was 2.5, 8.0 and 6.5%, resp.; 99.8% of the same population had antibodies against the subtypes current since their birth.

3. These illegitimate antibodies are, generally, not a subset of the legitimate antibodies: the fraction bound to and eluted from the extra-subtypic test viruses does not cross-react with representatives of subtypes current during the cohort's lifetime.

4. The illegitimate antibodies are not directed against the junior antigens we used as test viruses, nor do they fall within their hierarchic family. The low complementarity (i.e., flat endpoints and partial absorption) makes them comparable only to antibodies against bridging strains arising within that subtype. This point remains inferential until antigens inducing such responses have been isolated.

III   Conclusions

Since some observations, either in the field or in the laboratory, are more firmly established than others, the conclusions will also be graded, from compelling, through tentative, to purely speculative. They are listed here in order of decreasing solidity.

1. The first phase of a subtype, starting with the initial pandemic, is characterized by increasingly senior antigenic mutants.

2. Field strains are not purely antigenic mutants: many of them score as adsorptive variants and, judging by the peptide maps, are likely to carry also adaptive and gratuitous mutations.

3. Strains of the hierarchic phase, like the corresponding laboratory mutants, are not necessarily direct descendants of each other. The family tree may branch and may also form a network – it is degenerate.

4. The hierarchic phase is bounded: neither its terminal forms nor any of their predecessors have much chance of survival in face of a herd immunity which itself is increasing hierarchically. Strains of this phase are usually not isolated in the years following their appearance and, especially, not during the second phase of a subtype era.

5. Senior members of the hierarchic series are not the source of new subtypes. In the laboratory they behave as terminal forms, and in the field they are separated from the next subtype by an interval of 3-6 years.

6. The second phase of a subtype is multifocal, i.e., characterized by regional epidemics rather than monofocal pandemics.

7. Field strains of the bridging phase are not hierarchic. Each is senior to the first member of the hierarchic series, but not to the last and not to each other.

8. There is no uniform herd immunity against viruses of the bridging phase: similar strains may be isolated over the years in different localities or from different age groups.

9. Bridging strains are not well adapted (just like the corresponding laboratory mutants) but as can be judged from serological surveys, are omnipresent.

10. Immediately before the transition of subtypes, strains are current which actually bridge the old and new subtypes. Since back-mutants of such viruses represent the junior member of either subtype, bridging strains form a self-renewing reservoir of human influenza A.

REFERENCES

ARCHETTI, I. and HORSFALL, F. L. (1950) J. Exp. Med., *92* , 441.
BURNET, F. M. and BULL, D. R. (1943) Austral. J. Exp. Biol., *21* , 55.
BURNET, F. M., McCREA, J. F. and STONE, J. D. (1946) Br. J. Exp. Path., *27*, 228.
DAVENPORT, F. M., HENNESSY, A. V. and FRANCIS, T. (1953) J. Exp. Med., *98* , 641.
DAVENPORT, F. M. and HENNESSY, A. V. (1958) Ann. Int. Med., *49*, 493.
DAVENPORT, F. M., HENNESSY, A. V. and MINUSE, E. (1967) J. Exp. Med., *126* , 1049.
DAVENPORT, F. M., MINUSE, E. HENNESSY, A. V. and FRANCIS, T. (1969) Bull. WHO, *41* , 453.
DOWDLE, W. R., COLEMAN, M. T. and GREGG, M. B. (1974) Prog. Med. Virol., *17*, 91.

FAZEKAS DE ST. GROTH, S. (1962) Adv. Virus Res., *9*, 1.

FAZEKAS DE ST. GROTH, S. (1967) Cold Spring Harbor Symp., *32*, 525.

FAZEKAS DE ST. GROTH, S. (1969a) J. Immunol., *103*, 1107.

FAZEKAS DE ST. GROTH, S. (1969b) Bull. WHO, *41* 651.

FAZEKAS DE ST. GROTH, S. (1970) Arch. Environ. Health *21*, 293.

FAZEKAS DE ST. GROTH, S. (1975) in Negative Strand Viruses (Eds. B. W. J. Mahy and R. D. Barry, Academic Press, New York) p. 741.

FAZEKAS DE ST. GROTH, S. and TEES, R. (1975) Intervirol., *5*, 335.

FAZEKAS DE ST. GROTH, S. and GERHARD, W. (in preparation).

FAZEKAS DE ST. GROTH, S. and TEES, R. (unpublished observations).

FAZEKAS DE ST. GROTH, S. and UNDERWOOD, A. P. (1977) submitted for publication.

FRANCIS, T. (1952) Fed. Proc., *11*, 808.

FRANCIS, T. (1960) Proc. Am. Phil. Soc., *104*, 572.

FRIEDEWALD, W. F. (1944) J. Exp. Med., *79*, 633.

FUKUMI, H. (1969) Bull. WHO, *41*, 469.

FUKUMI, H. (1970) Arch. Environ. Health, *21*, 304.

HANNOUN, C. (1974) personal communication.

HILLEMAN, M. R. (1951) Proc. Soc. Exp. Biol. Med., *78*, 208.

ISAACS, A. and ANDREWES, C. H. (1951) Br. Med. J. *ii*, 921.

MARINE, W. M. and WORKMAN, W. M. (1969) Am. J. Epid., *90*, 406.

MARINE, W. M., WORKMAN, W. M. and WEBSTER, R. G. (1969) Bull. WHO. *41*, 475.

MASUREL, N. (1967) Ned. T. Geneesk., *111*, 1245

MASUREL, N. (1968) Nature, *218*, 100.

MASUREL, N. (1969a) Lancet, *i*, 907.

MASUREL, N. (1969b) Bull. WHO, *41*, 461.

MASUREL, N. and MULDER, J. (1966) Bull. WHO, *34*, 885.

MULDER, J. and MASUREL, N. (1958) Lancet, *i*, 810.

TAKÁ TSY, G. and FÜRÉSZ, J. (1956) A. Microb. Hung., *2*, 105.

TAYLOR, R. M. (1949) Am. J. Publ. Health, *39*, 171.

WORLD HEALTH ORGANIZATION (1977) WHO Wkly. Epid. Rec., *52*, 38.

ZAKSTELSKAJA, L. J., EVSTIGNEEVA, N. A., ISACHENKO, V. A., SHENDEROVITCH, S. P. and EFIMOVA, V. A. (1969) Am. J. Epid., *90*, 400.

THE HEMAGGLUTININ GENE OF INFLUENZA VIRUSES

Peter Palese

Summary

1. The gene order for several influenza viruses was established by identifying the RNAs and proteins of different influenza recombinant viruses using polyacrylamide gel and serologic techniques. Partial maps of many viruses containing the H0, H1, H2, H3 or Hsw hemagglutinins showed that gene (RNA) 4 always codes for hemagglutinin.

2. The ts defect of 7 mutant groups was identified by analyzing recombinants in which the ts gene was exchanged. One hemagglutinin mutant, ts 61S, which was shown by this technique to contain a single ts lesion (in the hemagglutinin), failed to synthesize fully glycosylated hemagglutinin molecules at the nonpermissive temperature.

3. Comparison of the RNA patterns of different swine viruses isolated last fall and winter from pigs in Wisconsin showed major differences in the hemagglutinin genes and in genes coding for nonsurface proteins. The RNA pattern of one swine virus isolated from man seems to identical with those of viruses isolated from several pigs.

Introduction

The genome of influenza A virus consists of 8 distinct single stranded RNA segments. This conclusion is based on the fact that many different influenza viruses contain 8 RNA species when separated on polyacrylamide gels (Pons, 1976; Bean and Simpson, 1976; Palese and Schulman, 1976a, 1976b; Ritchey et al., 1976; McGeoch et al., 1976; Scholtissek et al., 1976). In addition, 8 corresponding mRNA fragments were detected in influenza virus infected tissue culture cells (Pons, 1977). It is therefore unlikely that the observation of nine influenza virus RNA segments (Skehel, 1976) is a distinct feature for all influenza viruses. Rather it appears that additional RNA bands which are occasionally observed are the result of contaminating defective particles possessing RNA segments with deletions. Such additional RNA fragments have been observed in virus preparations grown at high multiplicity (Palese and Schulman, 1976a).

Genetic Map of Influenza Virus

The fortuitous finding of unique RNA banding patterns of two different influenza viruses permitted us to analyze the gene composition of many different recombinant viruses which derived genes from both parents. The two parent viruses used in our experiments were A/PR/8/34 (H0N1) virus and a more recent strain A/HK/8/68 (H3N2) virus. After mixed infection of tissue culture cells with PR8 virus and an ultraviolet light treated preparation of HK virus, recombinants were selected in the presence of appropriate antiserum to contain HK hemagglutinin and PR8 neuraminidase. These conditions favored the selection of recombinants, which derived most of their genes from the nonirradiated parent (except for the hemagglutinin) (Schulman and Palese, 1976). Analysis of one such recombinant revealed that only RNA 4 (counting the slowest moving band as RNA 1) was derived from HK virus and that all other genes were derived from PR8 virus, suggesting that fragment 4 was the gene coding for the hemagglutinin (Palese and Schulman, 1976b).

This experiment also clearly showed that the genetic information for hemagglutinin resides in a single gene and that the hemagglutinin gene can be segregated from the remaining seven genes of a particular virus. Although non-linkage of the hemagglutinin gene was suspected, experimental proof for this idea was demonstrated only after analysis of recombinants which contained seven genes from one parent and the hemagglutinin gene from the other parent.

Similar analysis of the RNAs and surface proteins of other recombinants enabled us to identify RNA 5 in HK virus and RNA 6 in PR8 virus as the genes coding for neuraminidase. Mapping of the genes coding for nonsurface proteins was made possible through the development of gradient polyacrylamide gels which enabled us to identify the derivation of all of the proteins in recombinant viruses (Ritchey et al., 1977). Simultaneous analysis of the derivation of RNAs and proteins in many different recombinants then led to the construction of a complete genetic map for influenza A/PR/8/34 and A/HK/8/68 viruses (Palese et al, 1977a; Ritchey et al., 1976). The gene product of each RNA segment was identified and except for the neuraminidase and the nucleoprotein the gene order is identical in both viruses (Table 1).

Subsequently we determined the gene order for several other influenza viruses which belong to different subgroups (Palese et al., 1976; Palese et al., 1977b;

Table 1
Genetic Map of Influenza Viruses

	Protein	
	A/PR/8/34	A/HK/8/68
RNA Segment	Virus	Virus
1	P3	P3
2	P1	P1
3	P2	P2
4	HA	HA
5	NP	NA
6	NA	NP
7	M	M
8	NS	NS

Ritchey and Palese, 1977). We found that the H0, H1, H2, H3 and Hsw hemagglutinins are all coded for by RNA 4, that most N1 and Nsw neuraminidase genes migrate faster than nucleoprotein genes and that most N2 genes move in position 5 (slower than the nucleoprotein genes) in our polyacrylamide gel system. The order of the remaining genes was the same in all viruses studied. Techniques involving analysis of recombinants derived from ts mutants (Scholtissek *et al.*, 1976) and cell free translation of mRNA fragments (Etkind *et al.*, 1977; J. Almond *et al.*, personal communication) were also used to assign protein products (HA, NA, NP, M, and NS) to their corresponding RNA segments.

An approach similar to the one described above can be used to map the genome of other segmented RNA viruses. Several laboratories are now studying the segmented genome of reovirus (A. F. Graham, 1977 Meeting of the American Society of Microbiology, New Orleans; B. Fields, personal communication) and of bunyaviruses (J. Gentsch, 1977 Meeting of the American Society of Microbiology, New Orleans) by analysing recombinant viruses which were derived from two distinct parents.

Identification of the Lesion in ts Mutants of WSN Virus

An extension of these 'genotyping' techniques permitted us to identify the temperature sensitive (ts) lesion in seven groups of ts WSN virus mutants which were first isolated by Sugiura *et al.* (1972, 1975). We have used the following approach to identify the genes carrying the ts mutation. Recombinants derived from the ts mutant and a previously 'mapped' virus were selected at elevated temperatures at which the mutant does not replicate and in a cell system in which the rescuing virus does not replicate. RNA analysis of the wild type (ts$^+$) recombinant permitted the direct identification of the 'rescuing' gene and therefore of the protein with the ts lesion. A summary of these efforts, which resulted in the identification of the defective genes in all 7 mutant groups and their correlation with specific functions is shown in Table 2. We found that P1 and P3 proteins are required for cRNA synthesis (Palese *et al.*, 1977b), that P2 and NP proteins are required for vRNA synthesis (Ritchey and Palese, 1977) and that a defective M protein most likely causes faulty assembly of virus (Ritchey and Palese, 1977). Mutants defective in the hemagglutinin (Ueda and Kilbourne, 1976) and the neuraminidase (Palese *et al.*, 1974) were shown by using this new technique to contain ts mutations in a single gene.

Table 2

Correlation of biological functions with specific gene products of influenza virus

Function	Protein	Mutant Group (WSN virus)
cRNA synthesis	P1, P3	I, III
vRNA synthesis	P2, NP	II, V
Attachment to cells	HA	VI
Neuraminidase activity	NA	IV
Assembly (?)	M	VII

Mutant Defective in the Hemagglutinin Gene

Previously Ueda and Kilbourne (1976) isolated a ts mutant (ts 61S) of WSN virus which is defective in the hemagglutinin. This mutant possesses a temperature labile hemagglutinin and cells infected at nonpermissive temperature with this virus do not hemadsorb. Protein gel analysis of cells infected at nonpermissive temperature by the mutant failed to reveal a hemagglutinin band in the position of the wild type protein (Ueda and Kilbourne, 1976). A more recent analysis of cells which were infected with ts 61S at permissive and nonpermissive temperature suggested however that the mutant virus does synthesize a hemagglutinin molecule at nonpermissive temperature (Ritchey and Palese, unpublished). As shown in lanes 1 and 3, Figure 1, after a 15 min pulse label wild type virus synthesizes at permissive and nonpermissive temperature a hemagglutinin molecule which migrates ahead of the hemagglutinin obtained after a 3 hr chase period (lanes 2 and 4). It is tempting to speculate that this is the result of incomplete glycosylation of the hemagglutinin molecule after a short

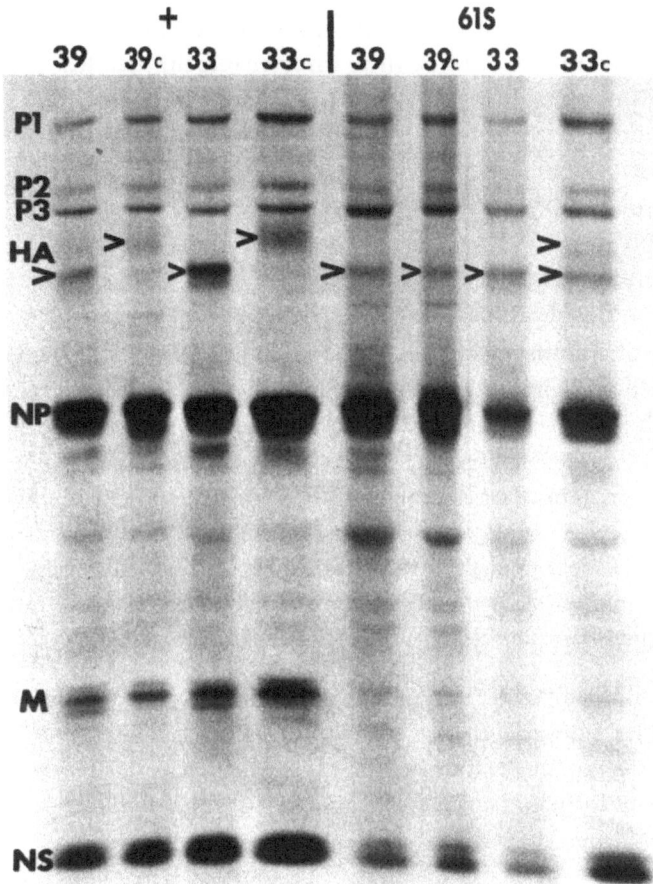

Figure 1

Protein analysis of cells infected with influenza A/WSN virus (ts$^+$) and its temperature sensitive hemagglutinin mutant ts 61S. Conditions of radioactive labeling with ^{35}S-methionine in MDCK cells and separation of proteins on polyacrylamide gels were described previously (Ritchey *et al.*, 1977). All infected cells were pulse labeled for 15 min at 6 hrs p.i.
Lane 1: Cells infected with ts$^+$ at 39.5°, lane 2: cells infected with ts$^+$ at 39.5°, pulse label followed by a 2 hr chase period, lane 3: cells infected with ts$^+$ at 33°, lane 4: cells infected with ts$^+$ at 33°, pulse label followed by a 2 hr chase period, lane 5: cells infected with ts 61S at 39°, lane 6: cells infected with ts 61S at 39°, pulse label followed by a 2 hr chase period, lane 7: cells infected with ts 61S at 33°, lane 8: cells infected with ts 61S at 33°, pulse label followed by a 2 hr chase period. Arrows identify the hemagglutinin bands after pulse label and after pulse label followed by a chase period.

pulse label. Cells infected at the permissive temperature with ts 61S show a protein pattern similar to that of wild type virus infected cells although less of the glycosylated product seems to be made after the chase period (lanes 7 and 8). However, at nonpermissive temperature (lane 8) fully glycosylated hemaglutinin of the mutant virus is not detectable, and no change in the migration of the polypeptide on gels can be observed following a chase period of 2 hrs. This result can be explained in several ways. First, mutations may be present in the mutant at or near the amino acids sites where carbohydrate side chains originate in the hemagglutinin molecule. Second, a mutation in one amino acid may change the secondary structure of the mutant protein in such a way that glycosylation cannot take place. Thirdly, it is possible that viral glycoproteins contain a signal sequence at the amino terminal (Blobel and Doberstein, 1975a, 1975b) and that mutations in this region change the posttranslational processing of the molecule. Preliminary protein sequencing experiments (D. Shields, G. Blobel, M. B. Ritchey and P. Palese) suggest, however, that the amino terminal of the mutant hemagglutinin is identical to that of the wild type excluding the possibility that the mutant protein contains an uncleaved signal sequence which could interfere with the correct processing of the molecule.

At this point the mechanism by which the mutant hemagglutinin fails to acquire the proper carbohydrate side chains at the higher temperature is not clear. Further experiments are required to elucidate this interesting temperature sensitive lesion and hopefully this work may provide us with a better understanding of the steps involved in the glycosylation of viral proteins.

Differences in the Hemagglutinin Gene of Swine Influenza Viruses

Comparison of RNA patterns of different influenza viruses has proven useful for studying possible relationships among recent isolates. For example, RNA analysis of the New Jersey 'swine' virus isolated in February 1976 at Fort Dix suggested that this virus was most likely not a recombinant derived from a recent human virus and an animal strain. Rather the RNA pattern of the New Jersey 'swine' virus resembled that of a swine isolated from pigs the previous year. The conclusion made was that the New Jersey 'swine' virus not only contains swine surface proteins but the genes coding for nonsurface proteins were probably swine-like as well. Based on the theory that new pandemic strains emerge through recombination of animal and human strains (Kilbourne, 1968; Laver and Webster, 1973; Webster, 1976) we then concluded that the New Jersey 'swine' virus was an unlikely candidate for the next pandemic (Palese and Schulman, 1976c).

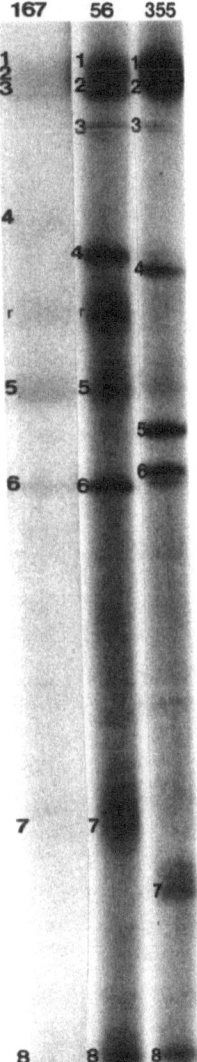

Figure 2

RNA pattern of three swine viruses isolated from pigs in the fall and winter of 1976.
Conditions of labeling and isolation of virus, extraction of RNA and separation of the RNA
segment on 2.6% polyacrylamide gels were previously described (Palese and Schulman, 1976b).
Lane 1: RNA of influenza A/swine/OM/167/76, lane 2: RNA of influenza A/swine/OM/56/76,
lane 3: RNA of influenza A/swine/OM/355/76. Some viral preparations are contaminated
with ribosomal RNA. 18S ribosomal RNA derived from the host is identified by r. In lane 3,
additional minor bands can be observed, which are most likely due to the presence of
defective particles.

In a follow-up on this study, we examined several other swine virus isolates obtained from pigs and compared them with the New Jersey 'swine' virus. Surprisingly, we found that swine viruses which were isolated in Wisconsin by Dr. B. Easterday in October and December of 1976 possessed highly variable RNA patterns. As can be seen in Figure 2, the fourth RNAs (hemagglutinin genes) are remarkably different in these three virus isolates. (In addition to the hemagglutinin gene, the other genes of these viruses also vary dramatically in their migration patterns.) This pattern contrasts with our observation that human H3N2 viruses appear to be much more homogeneous (data not shown). Confirmation of this latter observation, however, requires further analysis of additional isolates. Further experiments will also show whether or not differences observed in the migration of the hemagglutinin genes in swine viruses are also reflected in major antigenic changes, which can be detected by serologic procedures.

Comparison of the RNA pattern of the New Jersey 'swine' virus with that of another human isolate containing swine surface antigens, A/Wi/263/76, also revealed major differences in the hemagglutinin gene (in addition to differences in other genes). In contrast the RNA pattern of A/Wi/263/76 virus was identical to those of viruses isolated from pigs which were kept on the same farm on which the human patient lived (results not shown). This observation suggests that the same virus infected man and pigs.

Acknowledgements

This meeting report summarizes experiments which were done in collaboration with Drs. M. B. Ritchey and J. L. Schulman. I thank Dr. B. Easterday for providing me with some of the swine viruses isolated in Wisconsin. Work in the author's laboratory was supported by NIH grant AI-11823, NSF grant PCM-76-11066, and ACS grant VC-234. I also thank Ms. Marlene Line for her expert technical assistance.

REFERENCES

BEAN, W. J., Jr., and SIMPSON, R. W. (1976) J. Virol. *18*, 365-369.
BLOBEL, G., and DOBBERSTEIN, B. (1975a) J. Cell Biol. *67*, 835-851.
BLOBEL, G., and DOBBERSTEIN, B. (1975b) J. Cell Biol. *67*, 852-862.
ETKIND, P. R., BUCHHAGEN, D. L., HERZ, C., BRONI, B. B. and KRUG, R. M. (1977) J. Virol. *22*, 346-352.
KILBOURNE, E. D. (1968) Science *160*, 74-76.
LAVER, W. G., and WEBSTER, R. G. (1973) Virology *51*, 383-391.
McGEOCH, D., FELLNER, P. and NEWTON, C. (1976) Proc. Nat. Acad. Sci. *73*, 3045-3049.
PALESE, P., RITCHEY, M. B. and SCHULMAN, J. L. (1977a) Virology *76*, 114-121.

PALESE, P., RITCHEY, M. B. and SCHULMAN, J. L. (1977b) J. Virol. *21*, 1187-1195.

PALESE, P., RITCHEY, M. B., SCHULMAN, J. L. and KILBOURNE, E. D. (1976) Science *104*, 334-335.

PALESE, P. and SCHULMAN, J. L. (1976a) J. Virol. *17*, 876-884.

PALESE, P. and SCHULMAN, J. L. (1976b) Proc. Natl. Acad. Sci. U.S.A. *73*, 2142-2146.

PALESE, P. and SCHULMAN, J. L. (1976c) Nature (London) *263*, 528-530.

PALESE, P., TOBITA, K., UEDA, M. and COMPANS, R. W. (1974) Virology *61*, 397-410.

PONS, M. W. (1976) Virology *69*, 789-792.

PONS, M. W. (1977) Virology *76*, 855-859.

RITCHEY, M. B., PALESE, P. and SCHULMAN, J. L. (1976) J. Virol. *20*, 307-313.

RITCHEY, M. B., PALESE, P. and SCHULMAN, J. L. (1977) Virology *76*, 122-128.

RITCHEY, M. B. and PALESE, P. (1977) J. Virol. *21*, 1196-1024.

SCHOLTISSEK, C., HARMS, E., ROHDE, W., ORLICH, M. and ROTT, R. (1976) Virology *74*, 332-344.

SCHULMAN, J. L. and PALESE, P. (1976) J. Virol. *20*, 248-254.

SKEHEL, J. J. (1976) In: 'Influenza: Virus, Vaccines, Strategy', P. Selby, ed., pp. 111-119.

SUGIURA, A., TOBITA, K., and KILBOURNE, E. D. (1972) J. Virol. *10*, 639-647.

SUGIURA, A., UEDA, M., TOBITA, K., and ENOMOTO, C. (1975) Virology *65*, 363-375.

UEDA, M. and KILBOURNE, E. D. (1976) Virology *70*, 425-431.

GENETIC RELATEDNESS OF THE RNA SEGMENTS CODING FOR THE HEMAGGLUTININ OF DIFFERENT INFLUENZA STRAINS

Christoph Scholtissek, Wolfgang Rohde, Etti Harms, and Rudolf Rott

Two distinct types of antigenic variations have been described with influenza viruses: (1) the *antigenic drift* presumably is due to a number of successive point mutations of the hemagglutinin gene, while (2) the *antigenic shift* is thought to be caused by a recombinational event after double infection of a common host with two antigenically distinct influenza strains (for a review see Webster and Laver, 1975). In the latter case at least the gene coding for the hemagglutinin of the prevailing (human) strain should be replaced by the corresponding gene of the other strain presumably derived from an animal reservoir. The occurrence of such a new recombinant strain will then cause a pandemic, since no immunological protection will be found in man. The production of such recombinants is highly facilitated by the structure of the influenza viral genome, which consists of 8 single stranded RNA segments (Pons, 1976; Palese and Schulman, 1976; Bean and Simpson, 1976; Scholtissek *et al.*, 1976; McGeoch *et al.*, 1976). These segments easily can reassort in doubly infected cells and can give rise to a large number of different new strains.

Recently we have developed a method which allows us to assign the hemagglutinin to one of the 8 segments of the influenza genome (Scholtissek *et al.*, 1976). For this purpose we have labeled the virus with ^{32}P, and after purification and phenol extraction the RNA segments were separated on a polyacrylamide gel in the presence of 6 M urea (Floyd *et al.*, 1974) (see Figure 1). The individual RNA segments can be isolated and used for molecular hybridization with the complementary RNA (cRNA) isolated from the microsomal fraction of cells 5 hrs after infection (Scholtissek and Rott, 1969). In the homologous hybridization we obtained with all segments nearly 100% RNase resistance after heating and slow cooling under saturation conditions (e.g. Figure 2). If the cRNA of other influenza A strains is used for hybridization, the amount of RNase resistant radioactivity is in most cases less than 100% depending on the

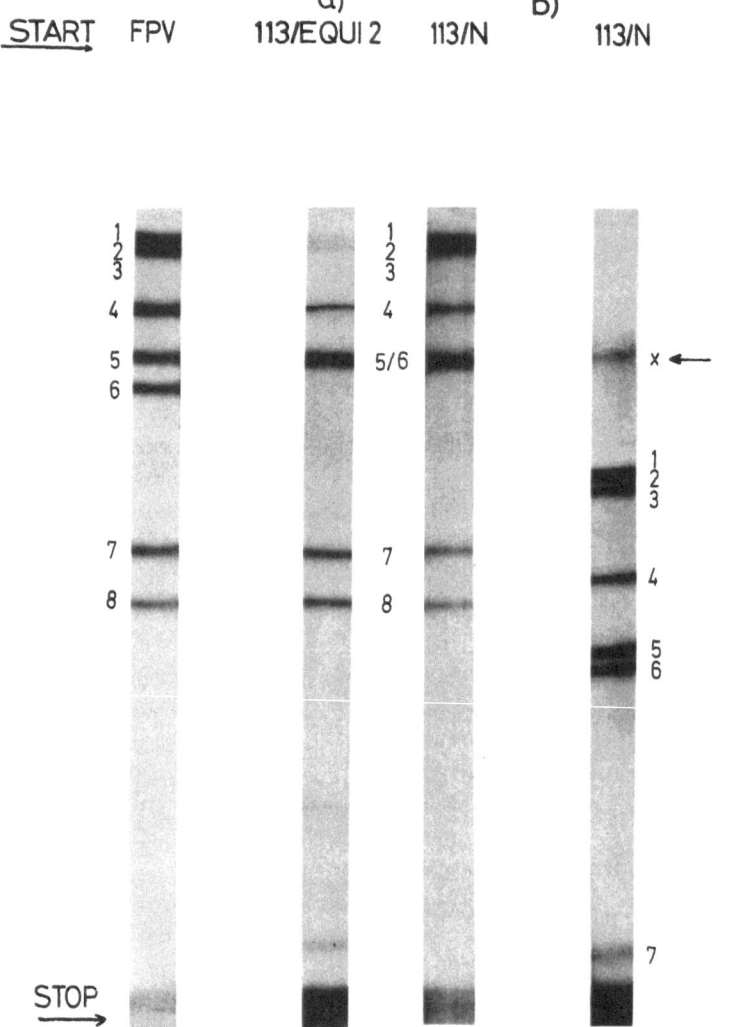

Figure 1

Comparative Genome Analysis of FPV, the Recombinants 113/Equine 2, and 113/N.

RNA samples were subjected to electrophoresis in a 2.8% polyacrylamide slab gel as described by Palese and Schulman (1976).

(a)   Electrophoresis was carried out at 30 mA for 24 hr at 4°;
(b)   Electrophoresis was carried out at 40 mA for 30 hr at 4°.

The recombinants have only the gene coding for the neuraminidase obtained from the rescuing virus. All other genes are derived from FPV (Scholtissek et al., 1976).

Table 1

Base Sequence Homology of Individual RNA Segments of FPV and cRNA of Various Influenza A Strains*

Non-labeled cRNA of	Base sequence homology (percent RNase resistance) ^{32}P-segments of FPV						
	1/2	3	4	5	6	7	8
FPV	100	100	100	100	100	100	100
PR8	50	63	34	76	73	85	87
FM1	51	65	39	74	78	85	86
A2	69	70	38	76	19	85	86
A3	62	65	47	78	19	85	83
Equi 2	56	66	26	75	19	85	81
Swine	58	78	37	74	82	85	86
Virus N	86	90	31	89	16	92	34
Dutch	81	90	100	95	65	94	95

*   For experimental details see Scholtissek *et al.* (1976). The following strains have been investigated: Fowl plague virus (FPV), strain Rostock (HavN1); PR8 (A/PR/8/34; HON1); FM1 (A/FM/1/47; H1N1); A2 (A/Singapore/1/ 57; H2N2); A3-Hong Kong (A/Hong Kong/1/68; H3N2); Equi 2 (A/equine /Miami/1/63; Heq2Neq2); swine (A/swine/1976/31; HSW1N1); Virus N (A/chick/Germany; Hav2Neq1); fowl plague virus, strain Dutch (A/FPV/ Dutch/27; Hav1Neq1).

genetic relatedness. Such values demonstrate to us the base sequence homology between the various strains. An example for the ^{32}P-labeled RNA segments of fowl plague virus (FPV/Rostock) is given in Table 1. Regarding segment 4, a base sequence homology of nearly 100% exists only between such prototype strains, which have an immunologically related hemagglutinin (FPV/Rostock and FPV/Dutch), while the other strains exhibit homologies of only about 30%. This correlation between serological and base sequence relatedness is a first hint that segment 4 is the gene coding for the hemagglutinin. A corresponding relationship exists concerning the base sequence homology to segment 6 and the serological relatedness of the neuraminidases. Thus this segment presumably codes for the neuraminidase.

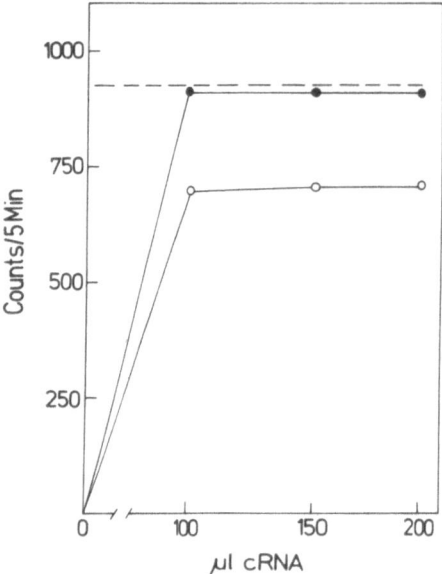

Figure 2

Hybridization – Saturation Curves of ^{32}P-segment 4 of Equine 2 and cRNA of Equine 2
(●——● and Hong Kong ○——○).
After hybridization overnight the samples were digested with pancreatic RNase. The dashed
horizontal line represents the input radioactivity.

A clear cut assignment of the various RNA segments to gene functions has been
obtained in the following way: first temperature-sensitive (ts) mutants of FPV
have been isolated and have been grouped into 6 recombination-complementa-
tion groups, of which the biological ts-defects have been determined
(Scholtissek and Bowles, 1975). These ts-mutants were used to produce specific
recombinants by double infection of primary chick embryo cells (natural host
for FPV) with other influenza A prototype strains, which do not form plaques
on these host cells. Thus both viruses singly do not produce plaques at the nonpermissive temperature; however, after double infection plaque formers were
obtained, which by definition have at least that segment carrying the ts-lesion
derived from the other influenza strain used for rescue. The cRNA of these
specific recombinants can be used now for the hybridization against the various
^{32}P-labeled segments of FPV: 100% base sequence homology indicates that the
corresponding segment of the recombinant is derived from FPV; less than 100%
RNase-resistance means that that segment is derived from the rescuing virus. If
the base sequence homology concerning a certain segment is high between FPV
and the other strain — e.g. segment 5 concerning virus N – the samples have to
be heated after hybridization in the presence of 1% formaldehyde close to the

melting point prior to RNase treatment in order to increase the sensitivity of
the method (see below Figure 3). In this way one obtains a clear cut answer even
with highly related strains (Table 2) and one does not need to rely on sometimes extremely small differences in migration rates of RNA segments or
proteins in polyacrylamide gel electrophoresis (Palese and Schulman, 1976;
Ritchey *et al.*, 1976), which, in some cases, are barely noticeable.

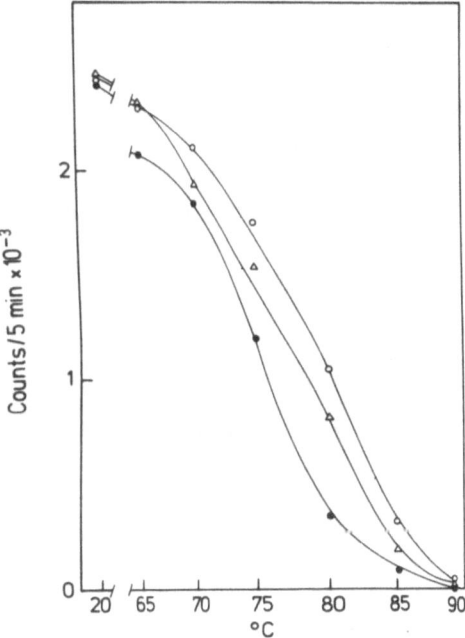

Figure 3

Melting Profiles of Homologous and Heterologous Hybrids of ^{32}P-segment 4 of PR8
After hybridization aliquots were kept for 10 min at the desired temperature in 1 x SSC and
1% formaldehyde prior to digestion with RNase (Scholtissek *et al.*, 1976).

o——o	hybrid PR8/PR8
△——△	hybrid PR8/WS
●——●	hybrid PR8/FM1

By the methods described we can (1) produce any kind of recombinants we
want, (2) we can analyze any recombinant by determining exactly which gene
is derived from which parent, and (3) we can assign genes to specific gene functions, since the ts-defects of our original mutants are known. The latter point is
demonstrated in Table 3: for example, if we start with the ts-mutant 3, which

Table 2

Base Sequence Homology Between FPV, Virus N and 19/N2

Counts/5 minutes after treatment with RNase*

cRNA	Segment number							
	1	2	3	4	5	6	7	8
FPV	4120	4120	4700	3720	5200	4600	3190	2360
Virus N	1980	2140	2600	1150	3560	860	1460	800
19/N2	3980	*2440*	*2580*	3700	*3790*	4560	3090	2280

* Segments 1, 2, 3, 5, and 7 were heated at 79° in 1% formaldehyde (Scholtissek *et al.*, 1976). 19/N2 is a recombinant between FPV-ts-mutant 19, which has a lesion in segment 5, and Virus N. The values of the segments derived from Virus N are in *italics*.

Table 3

Correlation Between Recombination Groups, Defects in Function of ts-Mutants, and RNA Segments of FPV

Representative ts-mutant	Defect in Function	RNA-segment	Gene Product
ts 3	RNA negative	1	polymerase 1
ts 90	transport defect	2	transport protein
ts 263	RNA negative	3	polymerase 3
ts 227	hemagglutinin negative	4	hemagglutinin
ts 19	maturation defect	5	nucleocapsid protein (?)
ts 113	neuraminidase negative	6	neuraminidase
-	-	7	matrix protein (?)
-	-	8	nonstructural protein (?)

has a defect in RNA synthesis (Scholtissek *et al.*, 1974), all recombinants derived from it have at least segment 1 obtained from the rescuing virus. Thus segment 1 codes for one of the two polymerase genes. If we analyze recombinants, in which the hemagglutinin is derived from the rescuing virus, always at least segment 4 is exchanged, indicating unequivocally that segment 4 codes for the hemagglutinin, etc.

The same method has been correspondingly applied to three other influenza A strains, indicating that in all four cases segment 4 represents the gene coding for the hemagglutinin (Scholtissek *et al.*, 1976; Rohde *et al.*, 1977; Scholtissek *et al.*, 1977). In Table 4 data are summarized on the base sequence homology of different influenza A strains concerning segment 4. It can be seen that in those cases in which a serological relationship exists concerning the hemagglutinins, as for example between the Hong Kong and Equine 2 strains, there exists also a relatively high base sequence homology. However, in cases where we have only little or no serological relationship concerning the HA we might have either a reletively low base sequence homology as in most cases or a very high homology as between PR8, FM1, and swine. There had already been doubts that H1-strains might emerge from H0-strains by an antigenic shift, since human strains isolated between 1934 and 1947 (H0) showed minor antigenic cross-reactions of their hemagglutinins to FM1 (H1) (Dowdle *et al.*, 1974). Furthermore, although no serological relationship between certain H0 and H1 strains was observed by the commonly used hemagglutination inhibition test (Davenport *et al.*, 1960), precipitin reactions could be demonstrated in immunodiffusion tests (Schild, 1970; Baker *et al.*, 1973). Our data make it extremely unlikely that FM1 is derived from PR8, and PR8 from swine by recombination, since these three strains are genetically not only highly related concerning segment 4, but also concerning all the other segments (Scholtissek *et al.*, 1977).

In Figure 3 the melting profile of the homologous hybrid of segment 4 of PR8 is compared with similar profiles obtained with heterologous hybrids derived from PR8 and WS or FM1 respectively. As can be seen all three profiles can be clearly discerned indicating that FM1 is somewhat less related to PR8 as compared to WS, which is like PR8 also designated as a H0 strain. In general, this technique should be sensitive enough to place a strain of an influenza A virus within the line of an antigenic drift.

It should be recalled that the genetic relatedness concerning segment 4 of Equine 2 to Hong Kong is only about 80% (Figure 2 and Table 4). This implies that Hong Kong is certainly not derived directly by recombination from Equine 2 (or vice versa), but that both strains might have a common ancestor concerning segment 4.

The ^{32}P-labeled RNA segments were hybridized overnight with saturating amounts of cRNA of FPV or influenza B-Mass, respectively. The values in the table represent the acid-precipitable radioactivity after RNase digestion. The input radioactivity is between 100 and 104% of the homologous hybridization. The figures in parenthesis represent the percentage base sequence homology.

We have also compared the base sequence homology of an influenza A (FPV) and B virus (B-Massachusetts). As can be seen in Table 5, there is a significant base sequence homology to all 8 segments of FPV. Concerning segment 4 it is

Table 4

Base Sequence Homology of ^{32}P-segment 4 of Various Influenza A Viruses to the cRNA of Different Prototype Strains

cRNA of	Percent RNase resistance after hybridization to ^{32}P-segment 4 of			
	PR8	Equine 2	FPV	Virus N
PR8	100	21	34	24
WS	99	n.t.	n.t.	n.t.
FM1	98	21	39	26
A2	32	24	38	29
Hong Kong	26	80	47	n.t.
Equine 2	24	100	26	31
Swine	85	25	37	26
FPV	31	26	100	37
Virus N	27	29	31	100
Dutch	n.t.	n.t.	100	34

Table 5

Base Sequence Homology Between ^{32}P-labeled Segments of FPV and cRNA of Influenza B Virus

cRNA of	Counts/ 5 minutes Segment number							
	1	2	3	4	5	6	7	8
FPV	1580 (100)	3180 (100)	1610 (100)	4370 (100)	4370 (100)	3630 (100)	1770 (100)	2080 (100)
B	600 (38)	710 (22)	380 (23)	1650 (38)	1900 (44)	710 (19)	910 (51)	880 (42)

38%. Furthermore, we wanted to know whether that part of the hemagglutinin genes which exhibits base sequence homology to segment 4 of FPV is the same in all these strains. This can be tested by mixing the cRNAs of the strains before hybridization. As shown in Table 6, the homologous part of the hemagglutinin gene of all these strains tested is the same in all cases, including influenza B, because after mixing the cRNAs no increase in RNase resistance is found. The same holds true for the neuraminidase gene (segment 6). Thus there seems to be a certain part of these genes which is higly conserved, while the residual part can vary considerably. The former part might be necessary for the function of the gene product, which is the same for all influenza strains, while the other part of the molecule, where we find a great variation, might be involved in antigenicity.

Table 6

RNase resistance of ^{32}P-segments 4, 6 and 8 of FPV after hybridization with mixtures of cRNAs of various influenza A viruses and of the influenza B strain under saturation conditions.

cRNA of	Counts/5 minutes		
	Segment 4	Segment 6	Segment 8
FPV	3920	3180	2260
PR8	1700	-	-
A2	2050	800	-
Equine 2	1950	810	-
Virus N	1930	790	990
B-Mass	1490	600	920
PR8 plus A2	2010	-	-
A2 plus Equi 2	2140	900	-
Equi 2 plus PR8	2060	-	-
Virus N plus PR8	2000	-	-
Virus N plus A2	2160	880	-
Virus N plus Equi 2	2100	880	-
Virus N plus B-Mass	2080	850	1040
PR8 plus B-Mass	1900	-	-
A2 plus B-Mass	2130	890	-

Experimental conditions as in Table 1.
· = not tested.

Since genetic relatedness is more meaningful and does not necessarily reflect the antigenic relatedness, it might be more convenient, or conceivable, to use genetic parameters on base sequence homology of all eight RNA segments — not parameters concerning the migration rate of the segments, which is rather meaningless in this context — to place the influenza A viruses into common subtypes. With regard to this parameter, the influenza A prototypes Hsw1, H0 and H1 would fall into the same group, while H2 strains would comprise a separate group.

Acknowledgement

The excellent technical assistance of Miss M. Orlich, Mrs. B. Homann and Miss H. Reincke is gratefully acknowledged. The work was supported by the Sonderforschungsbereich 47 of the Deutsche Forschungsgemeinschaft.

REFERENCES

BAKER, N., STONE, H. O., and WEBSTER, R. G. (1973) J. Virol. *11*, 137-140.

BEAN, W. J. and SIMPSON, R. W. (1976) J. Virol. *18*, 365-369.

DAVENPORT, F. M., ROTT, R. and SCHÄFER, W. (1960) J. Exp. Med. *112*, 767-782.

DOWDLE, W. R., COLEMAN, M. T. and BREGG, M. B. (1974) Prog. Med. Virol. *17*, 91-175.

FLOYD, R. W., STONE, M. P. and JOKLIK, W. K. (1974) Anal. Biochem. *59*, 599-609.

McGEOGH, D., FELLNER, P. and NEWTON, C. (1976) Pro. Nat. Acad. Sci. USA. *73*, 3045-3049.

PALESE, P. and SCHULMAN, J. L. (1976) J. Virol. *17*, 876-884.

PONS, M. W. (1976) Virology *69*, 789-792.

RITCHEY, M. B., PALESE, P. and SCHULMAN, J. L. (1976) J. Virol. *20*, 307-313.

ROHDE, W., HARMS, E. and SCHOLTISSEK, C. (1977) Virology *79*, 393-404.

SCHILD, G. C. (1970) J. Gen Virol. *9*, 191-200.

SCHOLTISSEK, C. and BOWLES, A. L. (1975) Virology *67*, 576-587.

SCHOLTISSEK, C. and ROTT, R. (1969) Virology *39*, 400-407.

SCHOLTISSEK, C., HARMS, E., ROHDE, W. ORLICH, M. and ROTT, R. (1976) Virology *74*, 332-344.

SCHOLTISSEK, C., KRUCZINNA, R., ROTT, R. and KLENK, H-D. (1974) Virology *58*, 317-322.

SCHOLTISSEK, C., ROHDE, R., HARMS, E. and ROTT. R. (1977) Virology *79*, 330-336.

WEBSTER, R. G. and LAVER, W. G. (1975) in 'The Influenza Viruses and Influenza' (ed. E. D. Kilbourne) pp. 269-314, Academic Press, New York.

ACTIVATION OF INFLUENZA VIRUS INFECTIVITY BY PROTEOLYTIC CLEAVAGE OF THE HEMAGGLUTININ

Rudolf Rott, Hans-Dieter Klenk, and Christoph Scholtissek

It is reasonable to assume that a virus disease is manifest in a clinical sense, if cells of vital functional significance are infected by the virus and are killed or at least modified by this infection. Since the tropism of a virus for a host cell represents primarily an interaction between the surface components of the virus and receptors of the cell it is appealing to postulate that structures of a virus surface might determine the infectivity and pathogenic properties of the virus. The results of our experiments have to be interpreted in this sense, because we could demonstrate such an inter-relationship for the hemagglutinin of influenza virus.

The hemagglutinin is synthesized on the rough endoplasmic reticulum and migrates via the smooth membranes to the plasma membrane. During this transport along membraneous structures the hemagglutinin is glycosylated to form a precursor hemagglutinin (HA) with a molecular weight of 75,000. This structure is cleaved into two smaller products, HA_1 and HA_2, which are held together by disulfide bonds (for reference see Rott and Klenk, 1977). Cleavage may take place either on smooth internal membranes (Klenk et al., 1974) or at the plasma membrane (Lazarowitz et al., 1971). The proteolytic nature of the cleavage reaction has been verified by the observation that in vitro incubation of virions with trypsin results in a conversion of HA to HA_1 and HA_2 (Lazarowitz et al., 1973) and that cleavage of HA in vivo can be blocked by a protease inhibitor (Klenk and Rott, 1973).

Proteolytic cleavage is not necessary for the formation of intact virus particles and for their liberation from the host cell. Under certain circumstances virus particles which still contain an uncleaved HA can be released from the host cell.

Particles with a precursor HA or the hemagglutinin composed of the cleavage products HA_1 and HA_2 are equally capable of a hemagglutination reaction, and in both cases the hemagglutination can be inhibited by specific antisera. This means that the reactive antigenic determinant is not significantly modified by proteolytic cleavage. The same holds true for the interaction of the hemagglutinin with the host cell. In all systems tested cleavage was not necessary to establish adsorption of virus particles to neuraminic acid containing receptors at the cell surface. A cleaved HA is necessary, however, for the infectious process to proceed further (Klenk *et al.*, 1975; Lazarowitz and Choppin, 1975).

Infection of embryonated chicken eggs or cells derived from the chorioallantoic membrane of the chick embryo with influenza strains of human and animal origin results in the formation of infectious progeny virus. Attempts to grow infectious viruses in chick fibroblasts are only successful with strains which possess the hemagglutinin of fowl plague virus (FPV), while all others have only a negligible infectivity. Analyses in polyacrylamide gels show a direct correlation between infectivity and the structure of the hemagglutinin. Only particles with a cleaved HA are infectious. A successful cleavage of HA which corresponds to productive conditions *in vivo* can be carried out *in vitro* by treating the inactive virus particles with trypsin. Such a treatment also activates infectivity (Table 1).

A productive infection of cells in which infectious virus is normally not formed is attained if trypsin is added to the culture medium. This becomes particularly evident, if cells are infected under single and multiple cycle conditions with a multiplicity of infection ranging from 30 to 0.003 PFU/cell (Figure 1). Growth curves of FPV which is synthesized in such cells as infectious particles with cleaved HA are identical irrespective of the presence of trypsin. On the other hand a clear requirement for the enzyme is observed in the case of virus N. When trypsin is present in the medium, replication is similar to that of FPV. In the absence of trypsin, however, newly synthesized non-infectious virus is only demonstrable under single cycle conditions. Under multiple cycle conditions virus production progressively decreases as the multiplicity of infection is reduced. This phenomenon also explains plaque formation by such strains which are normally non-plaque producers in chick fibroblasts in the presence of trypsin (Figure 2).

Whether a proteolytic cleavage is possible in a given host cell is determined primarily by the individual structural characteristics of the HA rather than by

Table 1

Effect of trypsin treatment on the biological activities of different influenza A viruses grown in embryonated chicken eggs or in chicken fibroblasts

	Rate of activation by trypsin of virus grown in			
	Chick embryo		Chicken fibroblasts	
Virus strain	Hemagglutination	Infectivity	Hemagglutination	Infectivity
A_0/PR8	1.0	1.3	1.0	27
A_1/FM1	1.0	2.4	1.0	4.3
A_2/Singapore	1.0	0.8	1.0	193
Equine 2	1.0	1.1	1.0	111
Swine	1.0	1.0	1.0	200
N	1.0	1.0	1.0	150
FPV/Rostock	1.0	1.0	1.0	1.0
FPV/Dutch	1.0	1.0	1.0	1.0

The virus particles were purified by density gradient centrifugation, treated with or without trypsin (10 μg/ml) for 15 min at 37°C and finally analyzed by HA and plaque tests. The activation rates are the ratios of the activities of trypsin-treated samples versus untreated controls. For details see Klenk et al. (1975).

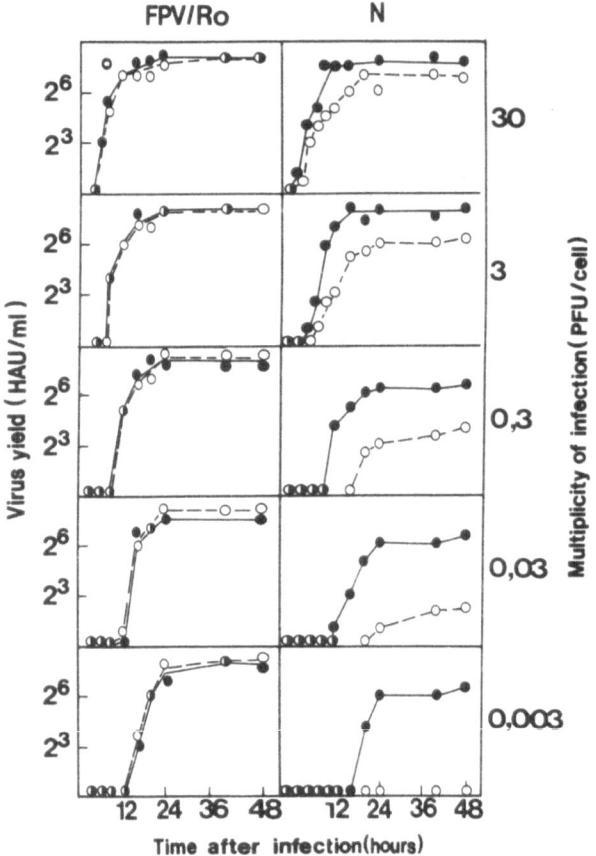

Figure 1

Single and multiple cycle growth curves of strains FPV/Rostock and N in chicken fibroblasts. Virus replication was analyzed in the presence (●————●) and absence (○ − − − ○) of trypsin in the culture medium (5 μg/ml). Virus released into the medium was assayed by hemagglutination. The inoculum was grown in embryonated chicken eggs. For further details see Klenk *et al.*, (1975).

the activation of cellular proteases by the infecting virus. This could be demonstrated by double infection of chicken fibroblasts with FPV and virus N, which are produced in highly infectious form or with reduced infectivity, respectively. Since HA_1 and HA_2 have different electrophoretic mobilities in FPV and virus N, it was possible to determine the origin of the cleaved HA in the mixed virus population by coelectrophoresis with homogeneous preparations of each virus. The glycoprotein pattern of the progeny virus is shown in Figure 3. The results

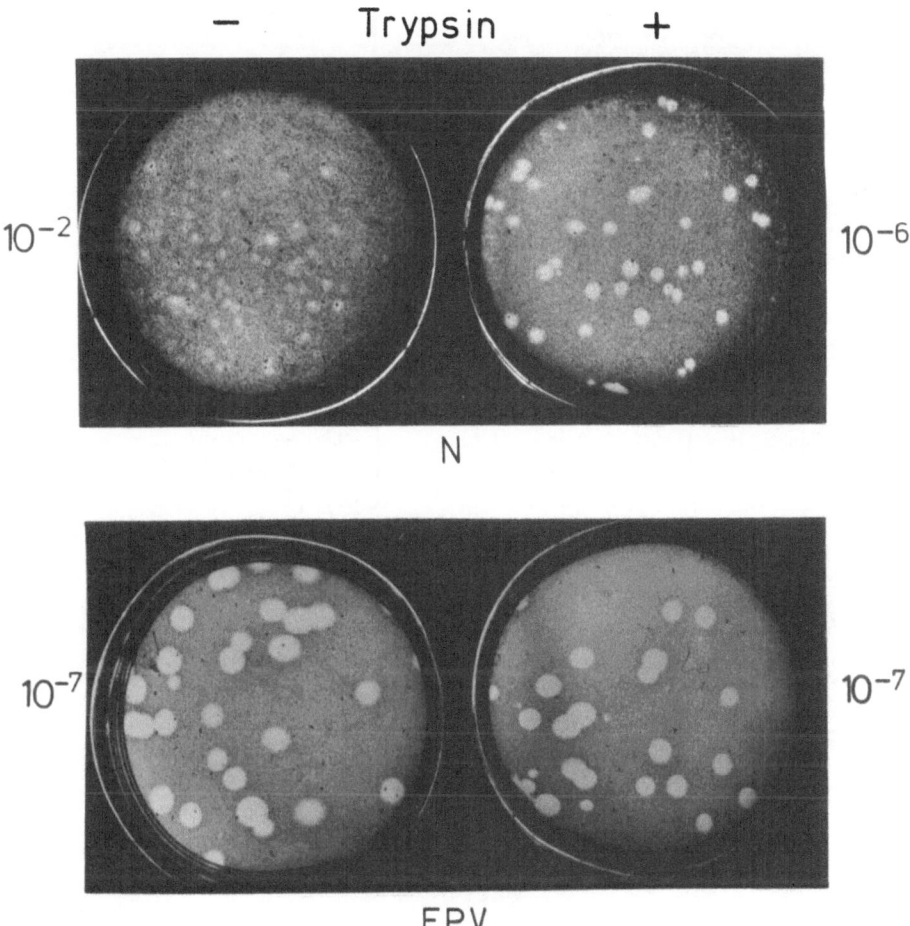

Figure 2

Plaques produced by FPV/Rostock and virus N in chicken fibroblasts in the presence or absence of trypsin (5 μg/ml) in the agar overlay. The cells were stained 3 days after infection.

show clearly that after double infection FPV does not induce cleavage of the hemagglutinin glycoprotein of virus N. Biological tests confirm our previous observation that virus N requires trypsin to undergo multiple cycle replication in chick fibroblasts, whereas FPV can do so in the absence of the enzyme. In doubly infected cells only FPV-specific hemagglutinin is formed if trypsin is absent. In the presence of trypsin, however, hemagglutinin of both strains can be detected (Table 2).

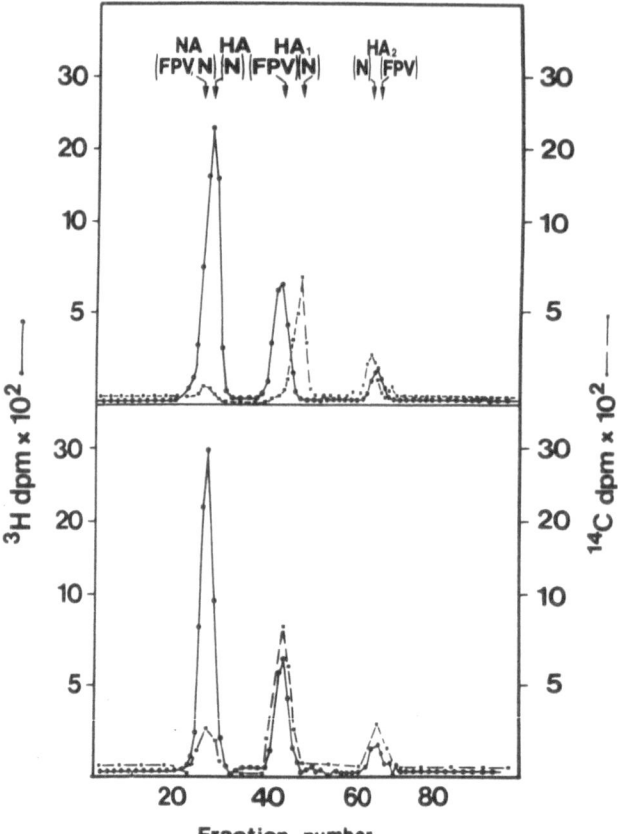

Figure 3

The glycoproteins of the progeny virus obtained after double infection of chicken fibroblasts with FPV/Dutch and virus N.

The virus was labeled with (^{3}H) glucosamine and purified. The upper panel shows coelectrophoresis with a purified preparation of (^{14}C) glucosamine-labeled virus N derived from chicken fibroblasts which was subjected to cleavage of the hemagglutinin glycoprotein. The lower panel shows coelectrophoresis with a purified sample of FPV/Dutch, again labeled with (^{14}C) glucosamine and grown in chicken fibroblasts. For further details see Klenk et al., (1977).

Summarizing these results it has been shown that the structure of the hemagglutinin itself decides whether a proteolytic enzyme of the host cell is capable of attacking the precursor structure which ultimately results in a cleaved HA which is necessary for infective virus particles.

Table 2

Effect of coinfection with FPV/Rostock on the infectivity of virus N grown in chicken fibroblasts

Inoculum virus (10^{-1} PFU/cell)	Trypsin present in culture medium ($10\ \mu g/ml$)	Yield (HAU/ml)	Progeny virus Specificity HI titer against	
			virus N	FPV
Virus N	-	2		
	+	128	4000	0
FPV	-	512	0	512
	+	512	0	512
Virus N + FPV	-	256	0	512
	+	256	4000	512

The progeny virus was harvested 24 hours after infection and identified by hemagglutination inhibition. For further details see Klenk *et al.* (1977).

To test whether formation of highly infectious virus requires cleavage of a specific peptide bond of the HA glycoprotein, we treated virus N grown in chick fibroblasts *in vitro* with a series of different proteases. Confirming and extending the observations of Lazarowitz and Choppin (1975) we have found that cleavage can be accomplished by a variety of proteases (Table 3). It appears that these enzymes attack different peptide bonds in the same region of the hemagglutinin glycoprotein, thus generating cleavage fragments of identical size. However, only cleavage by trypsin or a trypsin-like enzyme results in formation of highly infectious virus (Table 4). Activation of infectivity therefore requires cleavage of a specific peptide bond with arginine or lysine in carboxyl linkage. These findings suggest that highly infectious virus glycoprotein HA_1 has one of these amino acids at the carboxyl terminus. It was hoped that clostripain, a protease with a high specificity for the carboxyl linkage of arginine, might allow discrimination between these alternatives. However, such conclusions could not be drawn from our studies, since virus incubated with this enzyme showed very little cleavage of HA and no activation of infectivity. It should be noted here that our assumption that lysine or arginine are at the carboxyl terminus of HA_1 is not confirmed by the studies

Table 3

Extent of cleavage of the hemagglutinin glycoprotein of virus N by different proteases

Enzyme	Percentage of hemagglutinin present in cleaved form
Trypsin	100
Protease from Streptomyces griseus	100
Thermolysin	48
Chymotrypsin	45
Papain	34
Clostripain	15
Elastase	0
None	0

Virus was grown in chicken fibroblasts in the presence of (^3H) amino acids. The virus released into the culture medium was incubated for 30 min at 37°C with the various enzymes (10 µg/256 HA units). The virus was purified, and the amount of cleaved and uncleaved glycoprotein was calculated from the polypeptide patterns obtained after polyacrylamide gel electrophoresis (compare also with Klenk et al. (1977).

on the amino acid sequence of the hemagglutinin as it will be shown later in this meeting.

Plasmin does not cleave HA of virus N nor of a whole series of other influenza A (Klenk et al., 1975) and B strains (Lazarowitz and Choppin, 1975). Conversely, influenza strains which are readily cleaved in all host systems analysed do not require plasmin. Thus the essential role which this enzyme plays in the cleavage and activation of the HA of the WSN strain described by Lazarowitz and Choppin (1975) appears to be unique for this virus strain and probably reflects a peculiar feature of this hemagglutinin.

The observation that cleavage of HA is a prerequisite for infectivity but not for virus adsorption to the host cell shows that in addition to its role in adsorption, the hemagglutinin has an additional function in the infection process. It is presumably at the stage of penetration that cleaved hemagglutinin is required.

Table 4

Effect of *in vitro* incubation with different proteases on the infectivity of virus N derived from chicken fibroblasts

Protease	Virus yield, 20 h p.i. (HAU/ml)
None	⟨2
Trypsin	64
Trypsin + inhibitor	⟨2
Protease from Streptomyces griseus	64
Protease from Streptomyces griseus + inhibitor	⟨2
Chymotrypsin	⟨2
Thermolysin	⟨2
Elastase †	⟨2
Clostripain	⟨2
Papain ‡	⟨2
Protease from Aspergillus oryzae	⟨2
Bromelain	⟨2

Virus released into the culture medium of chicken fibroblasts was subjected to *in vitro* incubation with the various enzymes. The virus was then used for infecting chicken fibroblasts with a multiplicity of infection of 10 PFU/cell. 20 hours after infection the culture medium was tested for hemagglutination.

† The same result was obtained when the enzyme incubation was carried out at pH 8.6

‡ The same result was obtained when the enzyme incubation was carried out in the presence of cysteine (5 mM) and EDTA (1 mM) and in the absence of divalent cations.

For further details see Klenk *et al.* (1977).

Comparisons of the nuclear magnetic resonance (NMR) spectra of chicken fibroblasts exposed to virus N with either cleaved or uncleaved HA are being carried out in our laboratory by C. Nicolau and H-D. Klenk. The results suggest that the hemagglutinin is in fact involved in the penetration process. These studies indicate that virus N with cleaved HA induces an alteration in the fluidity of the lipid bilayer of the plasma membrane, whereas virus N containing uncleaved HA does not. Similar but more distinct fluidity changes have been observed when Newcastle disease virus containing a biologically active fusion glycoprotein has been compared to virus containing an inactive F glycoprotein. This could mean that the mechanisms of penetration process resemble each other in both cases and that the function, which is exerted by the F glycoprotein of paramyxoviruses must be attributed to the hemagglutinin of influenza viruses.

Since a hemagglutinin composed of the cleavage products of HA_1 and HA_2 is indispensable for the formation of infectious virus particles, only those conditions which have been defined in our *in vitro* studies can predispose to a pathological situation in the host organism. In contrast to former conclusions from others it is now clear, however, that viral **glycoproteins alone do not determine** pathogenicity of influenza viruses. **This could be convincingly** deduced from a series of experiments, where recombinants of fowl **plague** virus were compared *in vitro* and *in vivo* (**Rott** *et al.*, 1976). **In these** experiments there was no correlation between the presence of cleaved glycoproteins and the pathogenicity of the virus. **Furthermore**, using the same parent recombinants for double infection, the progeny back recombinants were only infrequently pathogenic for chicken, although they carried both surface antigens of the highly **pathogenic** FPV (Table 5). The results of these experiments show clearly that the pathogenicity of influenza virus depends on more than one gene. This conclusion was underlined by experiments (Table 6) **where** FPV recombinants were employed which carried a particular defined gene from other influenza viruses (Scholtissek *et al.*, 1977). Here again it became clear that the FPV derived HA cannot induce the disease in the natural host, but a certain gene constellation is necessary to make up a pathogenic virus. **Full** reconstitution of pathogenicity to levels of the wild type FPV largely depends on the parent strain being used for the gene exchange and the particular gene which is carried over. This means again that there is no individual gene coding for pathogenicity and that the HA gene is not a 'virulence' gene by itself.

At the present time we cannot list the optimal gene constellation to make up a pathogenic virus and we are not in a position yet to define the particular contribution made by the individual genes which might finally result in the complex phenomenon of pathogenicity.

Table 5

Pathogenicity of back recombinants for chicken

Recombination pairs	Recombinants tested	Activities of the back recombinants grown in chicken eggs			
		HA units	PFU/ml x 10^7	µg of NANA/ml	Pathogenicity for chicken (mean death time in days)
FPV(H)Equine 2(N)	FPV(H)FPV(N)	512	1.4	72	-
x	FPV(H)FPV(N)	512	10	64	-
Equine 2(H)FPV(N)	FPV(H)FPV(N)	256	80	206	-
	FPV(H)FPV(N)	128	36	152	-
	FPV(H)FPV(N)	1024	160	208	+ (3.5)

Taken from Rott *et al.* (1976).

Table 6

Correlation between RNA segment composition of recombinants and their pathogenicity †

RNA segment not derived from FPV	PR8	FM1	A2	A3	Equi 2	Swine	Virus N
1 (ts 3)	(1)○,○,■,○ (5)○,○,○	(1)●,● (2)●,■ (3)●,● (4)○,●	(1)■,●,■ (2)□,■,■, (3)●,■,○	(1)○,○,○ (2)■,,■ (3)●,,■,, (4)○,○,□,□ (5)○ (6)□ (7)■,,■,	(1)■,,■,,● (2)●,○,■	(1)■,,■ (2)●,,●,,■	(2)■,,■ (3)●,●,□
2 (ts 90)	(1)□,○,■,○, (4)□,■,○,■,■ (7)■,● (8)○,○	n.a.	(2)■,,■ (3)■,●,■	(1)○,○,○ (2)○	(6)●,●,,●	(1)○,○ (4)○,○,○	(10)■,,■ (11)■,,■

RNA segment derived from:

† Numbers in parenthesis are the numbers of individual isolates. Some of them have been described by Scholtissek *et al.* (1976). Each symbol represents one chicken. n.a. = no recombinant available.

■ means dead after 2 to 3 days after infection; ● means delayed death after severe illness;
□ means significant illness and recovery; ○ means no signs of illness;

81

Acknowledgement

These investigations were carried out in collaboration with **J.** Blödorn, E. Harms, M. Orlich, **W.** Rohde and W. Wöllert and were supported by the Sonderforschungsbereich 47 of the Deutsche Forschungsgemeinschaft.

REFERENCES

KLENK, H-D. and ROTT, R. (1973) J. Virol. *11*, 823-831.

KLENK, H-D., ROTT, R. and ORLICH, M. (1977) J. Gen. Virol., in press.

KLENK, H-D., ROTT, R., ORLICH, M. and BLÖDORN, J. (1975) Virology, *68*, 426-439.

KLENK, H-D., WÖLLERT, W., ROTT, R. and SCHOLTISSEK, C. (1974) Virology, *57*, 28-41.

LAZAROWITZ, S. G. and CHOPPIN, P. W. (1975) Virology, *68*, 440-454.

LAZAROWITZ, S. G., COMPANS, R. W. and CHOPPIN, P. W. (1971) Virology, *46*, 830-843.

LAZAROWITZ, S. G., COMPANS, R. W. and CHOPPIN, P. W. (1973) Virology, *52*, 199-212.

ROTT, R. and KLENK, H-D. (1977) in 'Cell Surface Reviews' (eds., G. Poste and G. L. Nicolson), North Holland Publ. Comp., Amsterdam. Vol. 2, pp. 47-81.

ROTT, R., ORLICH, M. and SCHOLTISSEK, C. (1976) J. Virol., *19*, 54-60.

SCHOLTISSEK, C., HARMS, H., ROHDE, W., ORLICH, M. and ROTT, R. (1976) Virology, *74*, 332-344.

SCHOLTISSEK, C., ROTT, R., ORLICH, M., HARMS, E. and ROHDE, W. (1977) Virology, in press.

THE STRUCTURE AND BIOSYNTHESIS OF THE CARBOHYDRATE MOIETY OF THE INFLUENZA VIRUS HEMAGGLUTININ

Hans-Dieter Klenk, Ralph T. Schwarz, Michael F. G. Schmidt, and Wilhelm Wöllert

Summary

Analysis of glycopeptides obtained after digestion with Pronase indicates that the hemagglutinin has at least two different types of carbohydrate side chains. The side chain of type I is composed of glucosamine, mannose, galactose and fucose. It is found on HA_1 and HA_2. The corresponding glycopeptide has a molecular weight of 2,600 suggesting that there are about 12 monosaccharide units in the chain. The side chain of type II contains a high amount of mannose and is found exclusively on HA_2. The corresponding glycopeptide has a molecular weight of 2,000 suggesting that there are about 9 monosaccharide units. The number of side chains per HA molecule appears to be in the range of 5 to 6. Host-specific variations in the carbohydrate content of the hemagglutinin are due to differences in size, not in number, of side chains.

Glycosylation of the hemagglutinin occurs in a stepwise manner. There is suggestive evidence that the core sugars (glucosamine and mannose) are synthesized in covalent linkage to poly-isoprenol and transferred *en bloc* from the lipid to the polypeptide. This takes place at the rough endoplasmic reticulum. After migration of the hemagglutinin to the smooth endoplasmic reticulum, glycosylation is completed by the attachment of the peripheral sugars (galactose and fucose).

The hemagglutinin spike of influenza virus is composed of a glycoprotein that is found either in the form of a single polypeptide chain (HA) or in a cleaved form consisting of two fragments (HA_1 and HA_2) which are linked by disulfide bonds and arise from HA by proteolytic cleavage (Lazarowitz *et al.*, 1971; Klenk *et al.*, 1972; Skehel, 1972; Stanley *et al.*, 1973; Klenk *et al.*, 1975; Lazarowitz and Choppin, 1975). The glycoprotein is anchored in the lipid bilayer by a hydrophobic segment at the C terminus (Skehel and Waterfield, 1975). The carbohydrate is present as side chains which are covalently linked to the polypeptide. Most of the carbohydrate appears to be attached to the HA_1 region (Laver, 1971).

This contribution is concerned primarily with the carbohydrate complement of the hemagglutinin. Our data are far from complete, so detailed structures of the side chains cannot be offered yet. However, I will be able to give some information on their number and size and on the problem as to whether they are homogenous or hetrogenous in type. I will then deal with their biosynthesis and will talk about studies employing glycosylation inhibitors.

The Structure of the Carbohydrate Side Chains

The studies aimed at the elucidation of the structure have been carried out on radioactively labeled and on unlabeled virus. I am not going to show you any data obtained from unlabeled virus. I would just like to mention that these studies clearly show, that the constituent sugars of the hemagglutinin side chains are glucosamine, mannose, galactose and fucose, and that galactose and fucose are present exclusively in terminal positions (R. T. Schwarz, B. Fournet, J. Montreuil, R. Rott and H-D. Klenk, manuscript in preparation).

Table 1

Metabolic Stability of Radioactive Marker Sugars †

Radioactive sugar used for labeling	Radioactivity recovered in original form ‡
(2-^3H) Mannose	80%
(1-^3H) Galactose	77%
$(1\text{-}^{14}C)$ Mannose	45%
$(1\text{-}^{14}C)$ Glucosamine	90%

†   FPV (Dutch) was grown in chick embryo cells in the presence of radioactive sugars and purified. The constituent sugars were analyzed as described in the text.

‡   Percentage of radioactivity present in purified virus. (From Schwarz *et al.*, 1977).

Incorporation studies with radioactive sugars can provide valuable information on the carbohydrate structure, provided that the markers are metabolically stable. Table 1 shows that not all radioactive sugars fulfill this requirement. Labeled virus was subjected to acid hydrolysis, and the constituent sugars were analyzed by ion exchange chromatography, paper chromatography and paper electrophoresis. The data show clearly that selection of the appropriate sugar

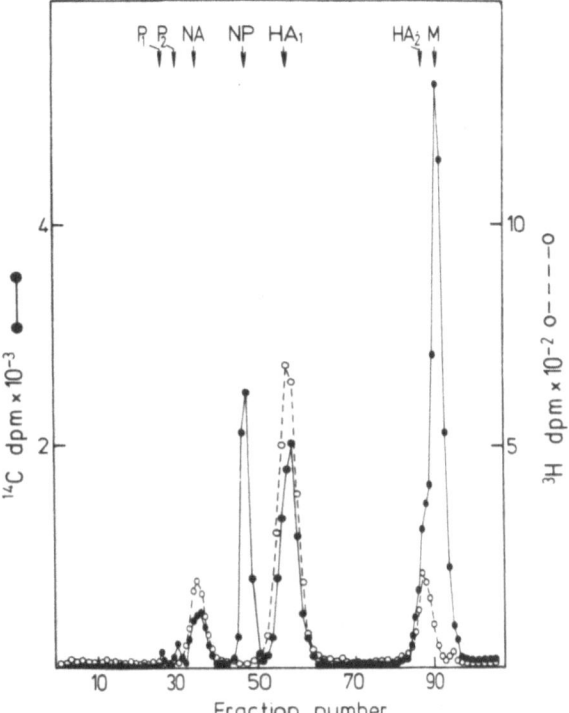

Figure 1

The polypeptides of FPV (Dutch) grown in chick embryo cells. Purified virions which were doubly labeled with (1-^{3}H) glucosamine (2 μCi/ml) and a mixture of (^{14}C)-amino acids (0.5 μCi/ml) were analyzed by polyacrylamide gel electrophoresis.

is important: e.g., (2-^{3}H) mannose is metabolically stable and, thus, a suitable marker, whereas (1-^{14}C) mannose is not, because only a small fraction can be recovered in the original form.

Most of these studies have been carried out on the Dutch strain of fowl plague virus (FPV). This virus has been selected, because all three glycoproteins separate well on polyacrylamide gels and can, therefore, be easily identified and isolated by preparative gel electrophoresis (Figure 1).

A standard procedure for the analysis of carbohydrate side chains of glycoproteins involves Pronase digestion of the polypeptide and subsequent purification of the resulting glycopeptide (i.e. the oligosaccharide plus 1-3 amino acids

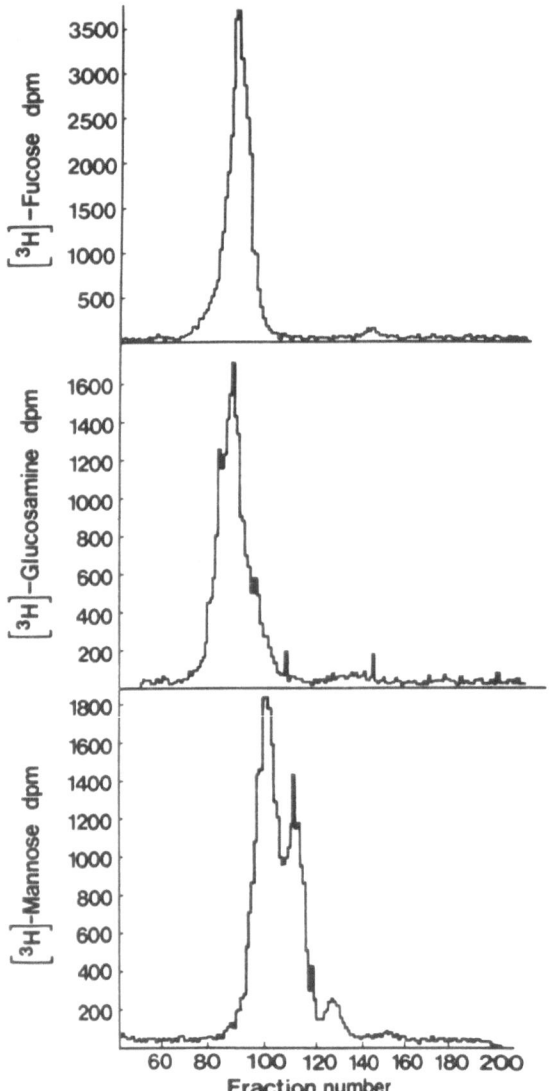

Figure 2

The glycopeptides obtained from virions labeled with $(1-^3H)$ fucose, $(6-^3H)$ glucosamine and $(2-^3H)$ mannose. FPV (Dutch) was grown in the presence of the radioactive sugars in chick embryo cells. Purified virus was subjected to Pronase digestion and chromatography on Biogel P6 as described elsewhere (Schwarz *et al.*, 1977). After labeling with fucose and glucosamine, only one major peak representing type I glycopeptide can be detected. After labeling with mannose, an additional peak appears at fraction 114 that corresponds to type II glycopeptide.

from the linkage site of the polypeptide). Figure 2 shows the glycopeptides derived from whole virus labeled with various sugars. By this procedure two types of glycopeptides can be detected. The first type has a molecular weight of about 2,600 and is readily labeled by glucosamine, fucose, mannose and galactose (not shown). The second type has a molecular weight of about 2,000 and can be discriminated only after labeling with mannose. Figure 3 shows the glycopeptides derived from the individual glycoproteins (HA_1, HA_2, NA) labeled with glucosamine. It demonstrates that type I glycopeptide is present in each glycoprotein. Corresponding experiments showing the distribution of type II demonstrate that this glycopeptide is found on HA_2, but not on HA_1 (Schwarz et al., 1977). This concept is supported by a comparative analysis of the incorporation of the constituent sugars into each glycoprotein which indicates that HA_2 is relatively rich in mannose (Table 2).

Table 2

Incorporation of Different Sugars into Influenza Virus Glycoproteins †

Radioactive sugar	Amount of label incorporated into		
	NA	HA_1	HA_2
(6-^3H) Glucosamine	16%	61%	23%
(2-^3H) Mannose	18%	40%	42%
(1-^3H) Galactose	18%	58%	24%
(1-^3H) Fucose	12%	70%	18%

†   FPV (Dutch) was grown in chick embryo cells in the presence of radioactive sugars, purified, and analyzed by polyacrylamide gel electrophoresis. Radioactivity has been found only in the viral glycoproteins, and the proportions present in NA, HA_1, and HA_2 have been calculated. (From Schwarz et al., 1977).

Since it can be assumed that the glycopeptides contain at least one and not more than two or three amino acid residues (Spiro, 1965), one can calculate from the molecular weights of the glycopeptides mentioned above that the carbohydrate side chains of type I and II consist of a maximum of 12 and 9 monosaccharide units, respectively. The molecular weights of the glycopeptides allow also a rough estimate on the number of side chains present in the uncleaved hemagglutinin glycoprotein of FPV. Since the total carbohydrate complement of HA was found to be 12,000 daltons (Schwarz and Klenk, 1974), the number of side chains appears to be in the range of 5 to 6.

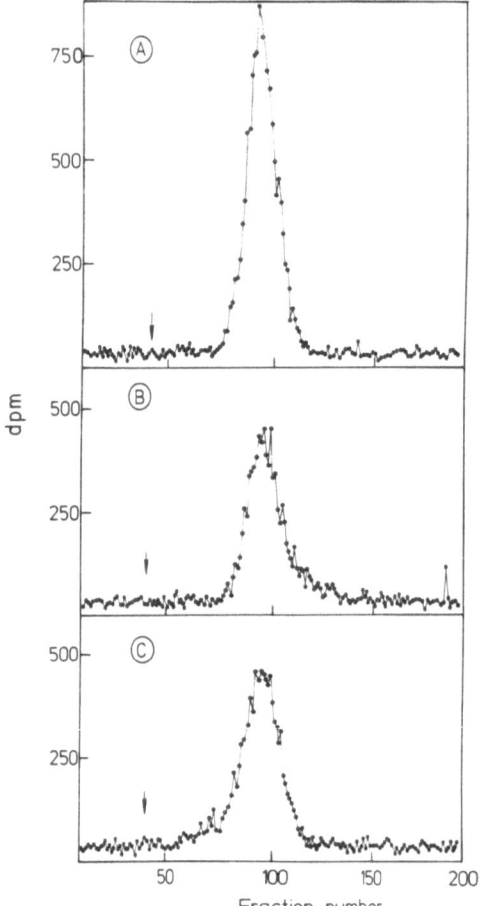

Figure 3

Glycopeptides obtained from individual glycoproteins of FPV (Dutch). Glycoproteins of virus labeled with (6-^{3}H) glucosamine were isolated by preparative polyacrylamide gel electrophoresis and digested with Pronase. The glycopeptides were analyzed on Biogel P10. (A) HA$_1$, (B) HA$_2$, (C) NA. (From Schwarz *et al.*, 1977).

It is a common concept that the carbohydrate chains in viral glycoproteins are synthesized by host-specific sugar transferases and, therefore, are susceptible to host modifications. Thus, the glycoproteins of influenza virus grown in MDBK cells have a higher molecular weight than those derived from chick embryo cells (Figure 4). Figure 5B shows that the difference in the molecular weight of the

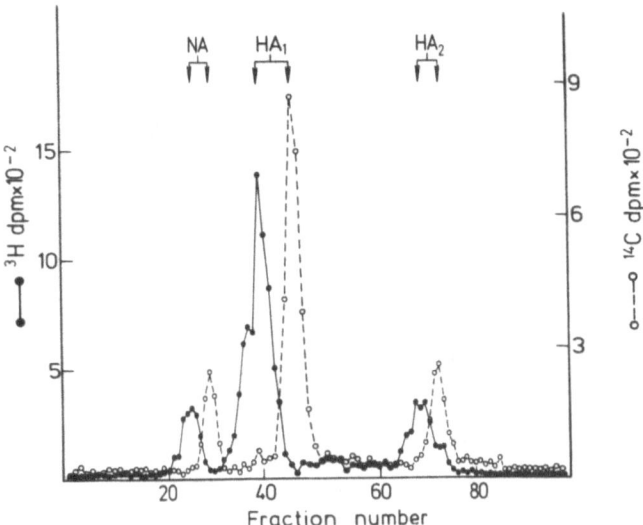

Figure 4

Glycoproteins of FPV (Dutch) grown in MDBK cells and in CE cells. Virus grown in MDBK cells was labeled with (6-^{3}H) glucosamine (5 μCi/ml), virus grown in CE cells with (1-^{14}C) glucosamine (1 μCi/ml). Purified preparations of each virus were mixed and coelectrophoresed on polyacrylamide gels. (From Schwarz *et al.*, 1977).

glycoproteins is paralleled by a difference in the molecular weight of the glycopeptides. This indicates that the differences observed with the glyco-proteins are due to variations of the size of the side chains rather than to vari-ations of their number. In contrast, different virus strains (FPV and Virus N) grown in the same host give rise to glycoproteins of similar molecular weight (Figure 5A).

The Synthesis of the Carbohydrate Side Chains

The synthesis of the carbohydrate side chains is intimately associated with the biogenesis of the glycoproteins and of the viral envelope, in general. Envelope assembly is a multistep process involving sequential incorporation of viral proteins into cellular membranes. A scheme of the sequence of events is given in Figure 6.

The scheme has been derived to a large extent from studies employing cell fractionation. This approach has also been used to throw light on the bio-synthesis of the carbohydrate side chains. The cell fractions were prepared

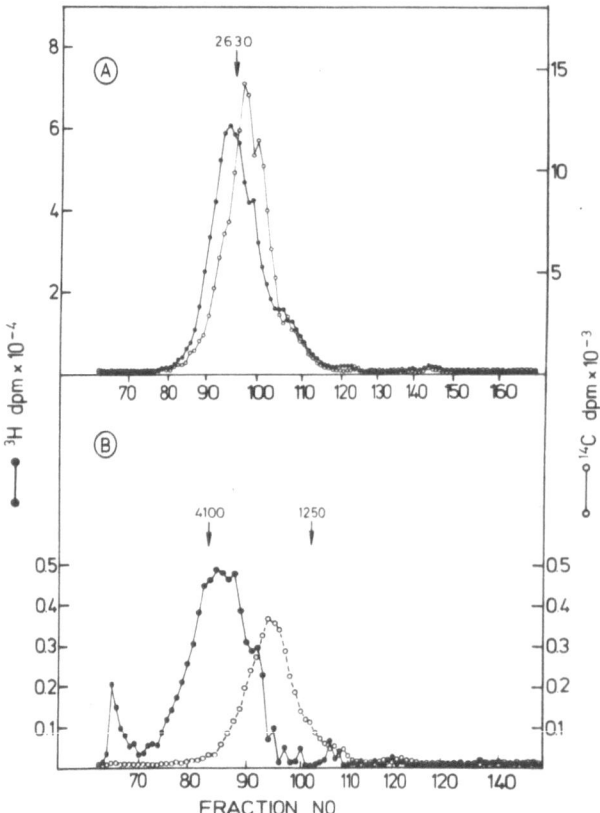

Figure 5

Glycopeptides obtained from two virus strains grown in the same host and from one strain grown in two different hosts. Virus N grown in chick embryo cells and labeled with (6-^{3}H) glucosamine was mixed with FPV (Dutch) labeled with (1-^{14}C) glucosamine and grown in the same cells (A). FPV (Dutch) grown in MDBK cells and labeled with (6-^{3}H) glucosamine was mixed with FPV (Dutch) grown in chick embryo cells in the presence of (1-^{14}C) glucosamine. The samples were digested with Pronase and chromatographed on Biogel P6. (From Schwarz *et al.*, 1977).

from cytoplasmic extracts by centrifugation on sucrose density gradients. It has been described previously that this procedure yields 6 to 7 fractions, and analysis in the electron microscope has demonstrated that fractions 2 and 3 consist predominantly of smooth membrane vesicles, whereas fractions 5 and 6 are formed by rough membranes (Compans, 1973a; Klenk *et al.*, 1974). Table 3 shows the distribution of marker enzymes specific for endoplasmic reticulum (glucose-6-phosphatase) and plasma membranes (5'-nucleotidase). Fraction 3

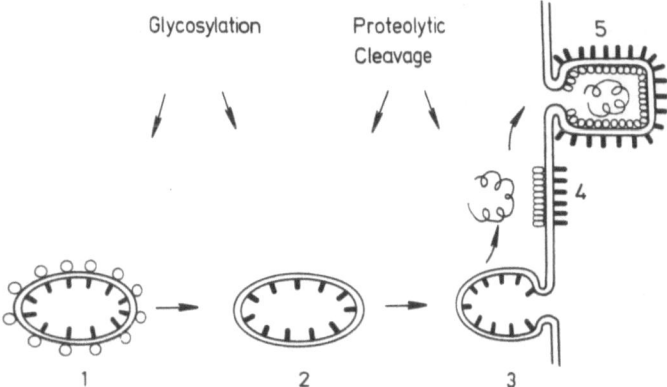

Figure 6

Sequence of events involved in envelope assembly. The polypeptide chains of the glyco-proteins are synthesized on the rough endoplasmic reticulum (1). From there they migrate via the smooth endoplysmic reticulum and the Golgi apparatus (2) to the plasma membrane (3). In the course of migration these polypeptides undergo posttranslational modifications. These involve sequential glycosylation at the rough endoplasmic reticulum (1) and at smooth internal membranes (2), and proteolytic cleavage which takes place at smooth internal membranes (2) and at the plasma membrane (3). The M protein attaches to areas of the plasma membrane containing viral glycoproteins. Thus, patches of viral envelope are formed which are able to bind nucleocapsid strands floating in the cytoplasma (4). The mature virus particle is then released by budding (5). (From Rott and Klenk, 1977).

contains a relatively high level of 5'-nucleotidase activity indicating that some of the material present in this fraction is derived from plasma membranes. However, since the specific activity was only about two times higher than in the whole homogenate, and since it can be assumed that the plasma membrane accounts usually for 5% or less of the total cellular protein (Neville, 1974) one can conclude that only a small proportion of the membranes in fraction 3 originate from plasma membranes. Thus, the data presented now confirm previous observations (Nagai *et al.*, 1976) by showing that the smooth membrane fractions prepared by the procedure employed here are derived predominantly from intracellular structures such as smooth endoplasmic reticulum (SER), whereas fractions 5 and 6 are derived from the rough endoplasmic reticulum (RER).

Virus-infected cells have been pulse-labeled with radioactive sugars, and the viral glycoproteins have been analyzed by polyacrylamide gel electrophoresis in fraction 5 containing RER and in fraction 3 containing SER (Figure 7).

Table 3

Amount of Protein and Marker Enzymes Present in Cell Homogenates and Cytoplasmic Fractions of Chick Embryo Cells Infected with FPV (Rostock).

	Cell homogenate	Fraction 2	Fraction 3	Fraction 4	Fraction 5	Fraction 6
Protein content †	-	4.8	13.9	8.0	10.7	21.0
5'-Nucleotidase ‡	0.563	0.367	0.623	0.569	0.273	0.089
Glucose-6-phosphatase ‡	0.228	0.843	0.477	0.717	0.238	0.322

†   Percentage of total cellular protein

‡   Specific activities (μM P_i/h x mg protein)

Glucosamine and mannose are incorporated already on the RER into the hemagglutinin which is found in this fraction still in the uncleaved form. After migration to the SER the hemagglutinin is cleaved. The glucosamine and mannose label is, therefore, found predominantly in HA_1 and HA_2. In contrast to these sugars, fucose and galactose do not or only poorly label at the RER, but show distinct incorporation at the SER. Similar data have also been obtained by Compans (1973b). They show that glycosylation takes place in a sequential manner, first at the RER and then at the SER.

These observations are compatible with the concept that galactose is present on the side chains in a terminal position. This is further supported by the observation that purified virus can be labeled in HA_1 and HA_2 after incubation with galactose oxidase and subsequent reduction with tritiated borohydride (Figure 8). Thus, in situ the enzyme appears to have access to galactose residues on both glycoproteins.

Valuable information on carbohydrate biosynthesis can also be obtained by studies employing glycosylation inhibitors, such as glucosamine and deoxyglucose (Klenk et al., 1972; Schwarz and Klenk, 1974). Another powerful inhibitor which has been recently studied in our laboratory is tunicamycin (Schwarz et al., 1976). If infected cells are exposed to increasing doses of glucosamine or deoxyglucose, the hemagglutinin concomitantly acquires higher electrophoretic mobility. We have shown previously that this shift in molecular weight is due to a gradual loss of carbohydrate, and that under conditions of complete inhibition the polypeptide chain of the hemagglutinin can be obtained in a form that appears to be practically free of carbohydrate (HA_0) (Schwarz and Klenk, 1974). When glycosylation was inhibited completely, we have not been able to detect particle formation. Under conditions of partial inhibition, however, virions are formed that contain hemagglutinin with reduced carbohydrate content (Figure 9). Instead of regularly shaped spikes, these particles have a fluffy surface coat (Figure 10).

To throw light on the mechanism of inhibition it was of interest to find out whether the reduced carbohydrate content was due to the incorporation of incomplete oligosaccharides or to the lack of entire side chains. Such an analysis has been performed on purified virus N which was grown in the presence of deoxyglucose and labeled with ^{3}H-glucosamine. Figure 11 shows that the mole-

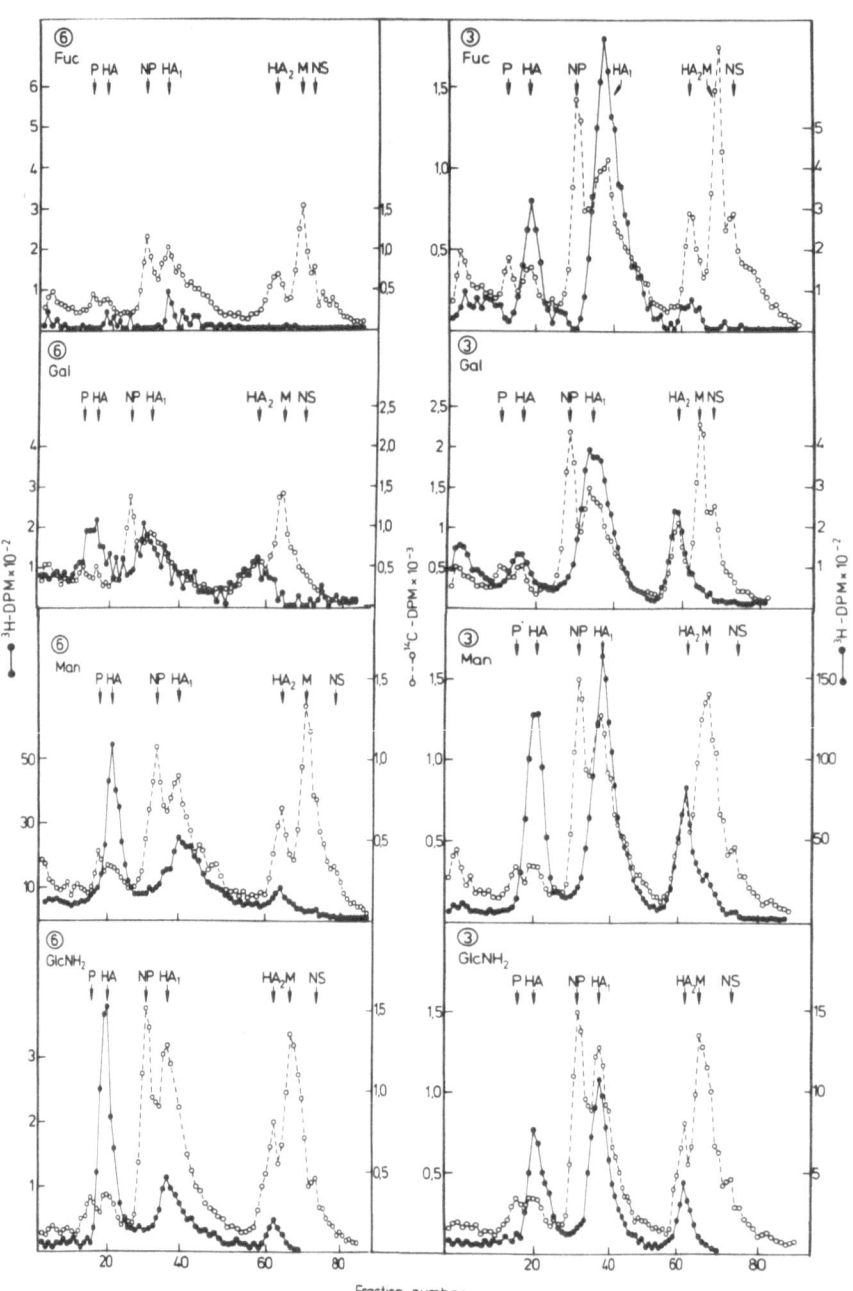

Fraction number

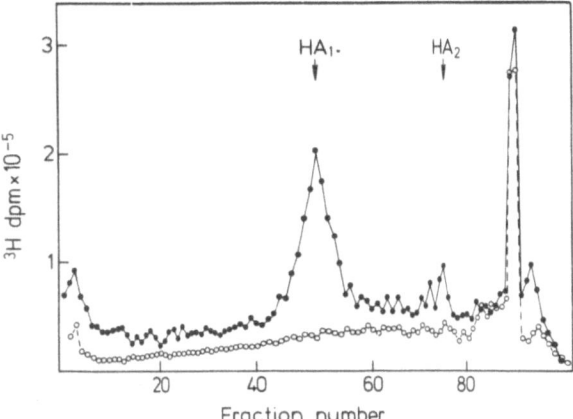

Figure 8

Surface labeling of viral glycoproteins by galactose oxidase and subsequent reduction with tritiated sodium borohydride. A purified preparation of FPV (Rostock) derived from eggs (10^5 HAU in 2 ml PBS, pH 7.0) was incubated for 3 hours at 37^0 with 30 μg galactose oxidase (Sigma, St. Louis, Ma). The virus was then repurified by centrifugation on a 10-40% potassium tartrate gradient (2 hrs at 25,000 rpm in a SW27 rotor) and dialyzed over night against PBS (pH 7.4). It was then incubated at room temperature with 2.5 mCi NaB^{3}H$_4$ (Amersham, England; 700 mCi/mmol). The reaction was stopped after 30 min by adding 1 mg NaBH$_4$. After extensive dialysis against PBS, the virus was pelleted and analyzed by polyacrylamide gel electrophoresis (●——●). Control virus not exposed to the enzyme has been analyzed on a separate gel (○ – – – ○).

cular weight of the hemagglutinin, which is present in the uncleaved form in this virus, is reduced if compared to that of uninhibited control virus. Figure 12 shows the glycopeptides obtained from the same virus preparations and from a preparation where glycosylation was inhibited by glucosamine. The data show that the molecular weight of the glycopeptides is not reduced in the presence of the inhibitor. Thus, it appears that the loss of carbohydrate is due to the loss of complete side chains rather than to a decrease of their size.

Figure 7

Association of the hemagglutinin glycoproteins with cytoplasmic fractions. 4 hours after infection with FPV (Rostock) chick embryo cells were pulse-labeled for 1 hour with either (1-^{3}H) fucose, (1-^{3}H) galactose, (2-^{3}H) mannose or (1-^{3}H) glucosamine, and subsequently fractionated. The cell fractions were analyzed by polyacrylamide gel electrophoresis. Viral proteins obtained by labeling infected cells 4 hours p.i. for 1 hour with (^{14}C)-amino acids were coelectrophoresed as markers. On the left patterns obtained from rough membranes, on the right from smooth membranes.

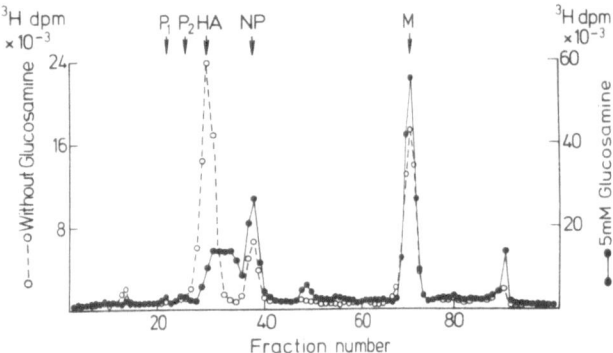

Figure 9

The proteins of influenza virions grown under conditions of partial inhibition of glycosylation. Virus grown in chick embryo cells in the presence of D-glucosamine (5 mM) and (^{3}H) leucine (5 μCi/ml), (^{3}H) tyrosine (5 μCi/ml), and (^{3}H) valine (5 μCi/ml) was purified by gradient centrifugation on potassium tartrate and analyzed by polyacrylamide gel electrophoresis. Control virus grown in the absence of glucosamine was analyzed on a separate gel. In this experiment virus N has been used which contains the hemagglutinin in the uncleaved form if grown under these conditions (Klenk *et al.*, 1975).

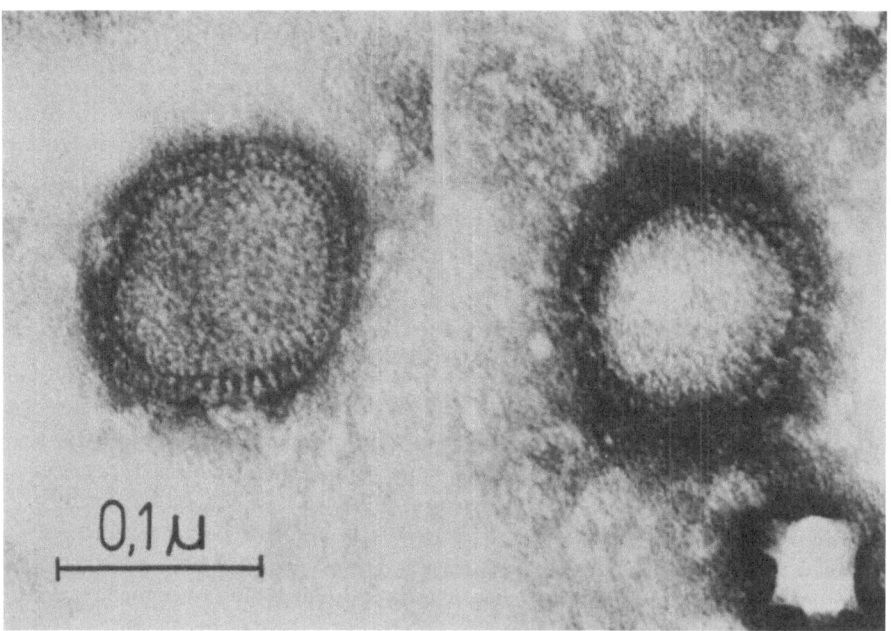

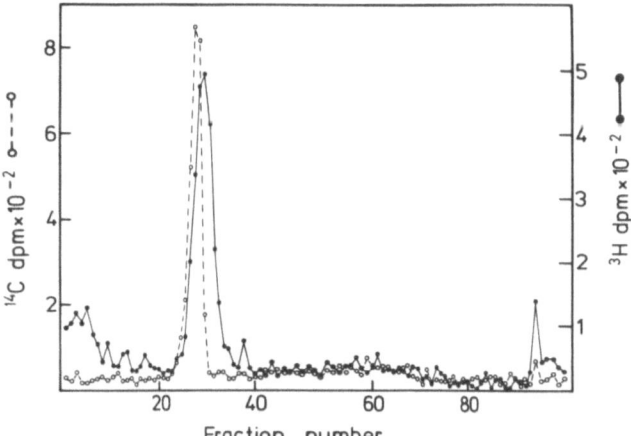

Figure 11

Glycoproteins of virus N under conditions of partial inhibition of glycosylation. Virus N was grown in chick embryo cells in the presence of (6-^{3}H) glucosamine and 2-deoxy-D-glucose (2 mM) and purified. Coelectrophoresis was carried out with uninhibited control virus labeled with (1-^{14}C) glucosamine.

This observation together with the above mentioned effect of tunicamycin allows several tentative conclusions on the biosynthesis of the side chains and the mechanism of the inhibitors. There is growing evidence that the cores of the carbohydrate side chains of glycoproteins are synthesized in covalent linkage to polyisoprenol derivatives and that they are transferred *en bloc* from the lipid to the polypeptide chains. It is known that formation of the sugar-lipid conjugates can be inhibited by tunicamycin (Takatsuki *et al.*, 1975; Tkacz and Lampen, 1975; Lehle and Tanner, 1976). The observation that this antibiotic interferes with the formation of influenza virus glycoproteins, suggests that lipid inter-mediates are also involved in the biosynthesis of the viral glycoproteins. Our data suggest that the glycosylation inhibitors interfere either with the formation of the oligosaccharide on the lipid matrix or with its transfer to the polypeptide.

Figure 10

The morphology of influenza virus grown under conditions of partial inhibition of glycosy-lation. FPV (Rostock) grown in the presence of 5 mM D-glucosamine (right) and control virus grown in the absence of the inhibitor (left) are shown. (Electron micrographs by Dr. K. Wahn).

98

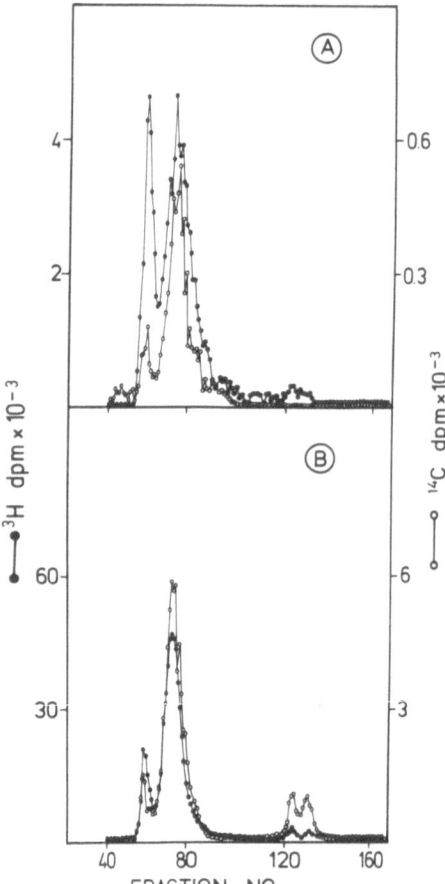

Figure 12

Glycopeptides obtained from virus N grown under conditions of partial inhibition of glycosylation. Purified preparations of virus N grown in chick embryo cells in the presence of
$(6-^3H)$ glucosamine and 2-deoxy-D-glucose (2 mM) (A) and of virus grown in the presence
of $(1-^3H)$ galactose and D-glucosamine (5 mM) (B) have been analyzed. Purified virus grown
in the presence of $(1-^{14}C)$ glucosamine without inhibitor of glycosylation was added as a
control. Both samples were digested with Pronase and chromatographed on Biogel P4. (From
Schwarz *et al.*, 1977).

Acknowledgements

The authors thank Frl. E. Otto, Frl. T. Islei and Fr. J. Winkler for expert technical assistance
and Dr. R. Rott for continuous support and many stimulating discussions.

This work was supported by the Deutsche Forschungsgemeinschaft (Sonderforschungsbereich 47).

REFERENCES

COMPANS, R. W. (1973a) Virology, *51*, 56-70.

COMPANS, R. W. (1973b) Virology, *55*, 541-545.

KLENK, H-D., SCHOLTISSEK, C. and ROTT, R. (1972) Virology, *49*, 723-734.

KLENK, H-D., WÖLLERT, W., ROTT, R., and SCHOLTISSEK, C. (1974) Virology, *57*, 28-41.

KLENK, H-D., ROTT, R., ORLICH, M. and BLÖDORN, J. (1975) Virology, *68*, 426-439.

LAVER, W. G. (1971) Virology, *45*, 275-288.

LAZAROWITZ, S. G. and CHOPPIN, P. W. (1975) Virology, *68*, 440-454.

LAZAROWITZ, S. G., COMPANS, R. W. and CHOPPIN, P. W. (1971) Virology, *46*, 830-843.

LEHLE, L. and TANNER, W. (1976) FEBS-Letters, *71*, 167-170.

NAGAI, Y., OGURA, H. and KLENK, H-D. (1976) Virology, *69*, 523-538.

NEVILLE, D. M. Jr. (1974) in 'Proceedings of the International Workshop on Cell Surfaces and Malignancy' Fogarty International Centre, Bethesda, Maryland, U.S.A.

ROTT, R. and KLENK, H-D. (1977) in 'Virus Infection and the Cell Surface' Cell Surface Reviews, Vol. 2, (G. Poste and G. L. Nicolson, Eds.) Elsevier, North-Holland.

SCHWARZ, R. T. and KLENK, H-D. (1974) J. Virol., *14*, 1023-1034.

SCHWARZ, R. T., ROHRSCHNEIDER, J. M. and SCHMIDT, M. F. G. (1976) J. Virol., *19*, 782-791.

SCHWARZ, R. T., SCHMIDT, M. F. G., ANWER, U. and KLENK, H-D. (1977) J. Virol., in press.

SKEHEL, J. J. (1972) Virology, *49*, 23-36.

SKEHEL, J. J. and WATERFIELD, M. D. (1975) Proc. Nat. Acad. Sci. U.S.A., *72*, 93-97.

SPIRO, R. G. (1965) J. Biol. Chem. *240*, 1603-1610.

STANLEY, P., GANDHI, S. S. and WHITE, D. O. (1973) Virology, *53*, 92-106.

TAKATSUKI, A., KHONO, K. and TAMURA, G. (1975) Agr. Biol. Chem., *39*, 2089-2091.

TKACZ, J. S. and LAMPEN, J. O. (1975) Biochem. Biophys. Res. Comm., *65*, 248-257.

INTERACTION OF INFLUENZA VIRIONS WITH RECEPTORS ON HOST CELLS AND ON ERYTHROCYTES

M. Vijaya Lakshmi, Chi-Lui Der, and Irene T. Schulze

It is well established that the hemagglutinin spikes on the surface of the influenza virus particles are responsible for the attachment of the virions to erythrocytes as well as to cells which support virus replication. It is also well established that the hemagglutinin receptors on erythrocytes from different species contain sialylated glycoproteins and that removal of the sialic acid residues from these molecules destroys their receptor activity. Although the virion receptors on the cells which are susceptible to infection (host cells) have not been characterized, it is assumed that sialylated molecules constitute the influenza virus receptors on these cells as well as on erythrocytes. However, receptors on host cells can be expected to differ significantly from those on erythrocytes. The major human erythrocyte glycoprotein has an unusually high sialic acid content (some 28% of its dry weight is sialic acid) (Winzler, 1969) and constitutes a larger fraction of the total membrane protein than does any single glycoprotein in other plasma membranes (see Hughes, 1973). In addition, whereas neuraminidase removes virtually all sialic acid residues from the erythrocyte membrane, some of these residues on the membranes of other cells are inaccessible to this enzyme (Eylar et al., 1962; Glick et al., 1970). Thus, a variety of glycoproteins as well as glycolipids could contribute to the hemagglutinin receptor activity of cells which can support influenza virus replication.

Although one might expect different affinities depending on the nature of these receptors on erythrocytes and on host cells, it is generally assumed that all infectious influenza virions are capable of binding to and agglutinating erythrocytes. Indeed, the use of infectivity to hemagglutinating activity ratios to measure the infectious quality of influenza virus populations is based on the assumption that infectious, as well as genetically deficient particles, have on their surfaces hemagglutinin molecules which are capable of binding to receptors on both erythrocytes and host cells. In these measurements, aggregation of erythrocytes is taken to be a measure of the capacity of virions to bind to cells. Conversely, failure of virus to agglutinate erythrocytes in the presence of soluble glycoproteins is thought to be due to binding of the virus to these glycoproteins instead of to erythrocytes.

Techniques are now available by which small and specific modifications in the viral hemagglutinin can be made. These involve changes in both the proteins and carbohydrate moieties of the molecules, and are known to alter both the hemagglutinating activity and the infectivity of influenza virus populations. Changes in either of these two activities can occur independent of the other, indicating that either binding *per se* or some step subsequent to binding has been altered. For example, we have previously reported that covalent attachment of sialic acid residues to the hemagglutinin of influenza has opposite effects on infectivity and hemagglutination (Schulze, 1975a; Lakshmi *et al.*, 1976). In addition, we have observed that fetuin, a sialylated glycoprotein, which inhibits hemagglutination, enhances the infectivity of influenza virus preparations even when the particles are devoid of neuraminidase. We have now used these systems to investigate the interaction of these viruses with both erythrocytes and host cells. Our aim has been to determine those properties of both virions and cell receptors which are important for attachment and penetration. The current status of this research is briefly described here.

The Properties of Sialylated Influenza Virions

Virions of the myxovirus and paramyxovirus groups have virion-coded neuraminidase on their surfaces and contain envelopes which are devoid of sialic acid (Klenk and Choppin, 1970; Klenk *et al.*, 1970a,b). Since erythrocyte receptors for these virions contain sialylated glycoproteins, we originally postulated that the function of the viral neuraminidase was to keep the virions free of sialic acid (Schulze, 1975a). Accordingly, we suggested that were sialic acid to be added to the virions, they would no longer be infectious because they could not bind to appropriate receptors. To test this hypothesis, we sialylated influenza virions *in vitro* using a soluble sialyltransferase from colostrum (Bartholomew and Jourdian, 1966) and demonstrated that, concomitant with the addition of sialic acid to the hemagglutinin, the hemagglutinating activity of the particles was indeed destroyed (Schulze, 1975a). Paradoxically, such virus preparations remain infectious and, under certain conditions, show enhanced ability to induce plaque formation. In an attempt to investigate these apparently divergent effects, we have undertaken to characterize the sialylated virions and to investigate their interactions with both erythrocytes and host cells.

Following overnight incubation with sialyltransferase and ^{14}C-CMP-sialic acid, some 2500 residues could be attached to virions from which the neuraminidase had been removed by mild trypsin treatment (Lakshmi and Schulze, 1977). When neuraminidase was left on the virus, approximately 1500 residues were added to the hemagglutinin. The amount of ^{14}C-sialic acid covalently linked to the two hemagglutinin subunits, HA_1 and HA_2, was then compared after different periods of incubation. The two glycopeptides were sialylated with about 5 times as many residues being attached to HA_1 as to HA_2. Since the enzyme used transfers sialic acid residues to terminal galactoses on glycoproteins (Bartholomew and Jourdian, 1966), we can conclude that after the virion is assembled, HA_1 has more galactose residues available for sialylation than does HA_2. These results are in keeping with earlier evidence that HA_1 contains 5 times as much glucosamine as does HA_2 (Laver, 1971), and support the conclusion that HA_1, the part of the hemagglutinin which must function in an aqueous environment, is more heavily glycosylated than is HA_2, the region by which the spike attaches to the viral lipid.

Following extensive sialylation, some 6 to 8 sialic acid residues are apparently added to each hemagglutinin spike. Preliminary experiments show that the isoelectric point of such virions is drastically reduced; sialylated virions are still negatively charged at pH 4.0 whereas the pI of control virus is 6.0 to 6.5.

Neuraminidase Activity of Sialylated Virions

Given this drastic difference in the charge properties of the sialylated and non-sialylated virions, we expected their neuraminidase activities to differ, especially when large substrates such as sialylated glycoproteins were used. We therefore compared the ability of sialylated and control virus to release sialic acid from two substrates, sialylactose (MW 633) and fetuin (MW 48,400) (Lakshmi and Schulze, 1977). Sialylation of the virus did not change its ability to cleave either substrate. In all experiments, the release of sialic acid from both substrates was linear from the beginning of the reaction, indicating that the viral neuraminidase did not have to remove sialic acid residues from the sialylated virus before it could efficiently bind either substrate. Neuraminidase assays were carried out at pH6.0; at this pH sialylated and native virus preparations differ vastly in charge properties. The experiments suggest that the hemagglutinin and neuraminidase spikes function quite independently on the surface of the virus and that the charge properties of the hemagglutinin do not alter the accessibility of the enzyme to its substrate. The observations are in complete agreement with the earlier conclusion that the hemagglutinin and neuraminidase fill only about one fifth of the volume of the spike layer (Schulze, 1972, 1973).

Since the neuraminidase activity was unaltered by sialylation, when optimum conditions for viral neuraminidase activity were established, the endogenous enzyme could remove the sialic acid from the virions and restore hemagglutinating activity (Schulze, 1975a).

Enhancement of Infectivity by Sialylation

Contrary to what we expected from the hemagglutination data, we found that sialylation of the hemagglutinin did not destroy infectivity; rather, the infectivity was either unchanged or enhanced as compared to that of native virions. With virions grown in chick embryo fibroblasts, enhancement was much more pronounced when infectivity was measured by plaque assay on bovine kidney (MDBK) cells (Madin and Darby, 1958) instead of on chick embryo fibroblasts (CEF). Following mild trypsinization which removes neuraminidase (Schulze, 1970) and cleaves any HA which is present on the virion to HA_1 and HA_2 (Lazarowitz et al., 1971), sialylation induced neither enhancement nor loss of infectivity although the hemagglutinating activity was destroyed.

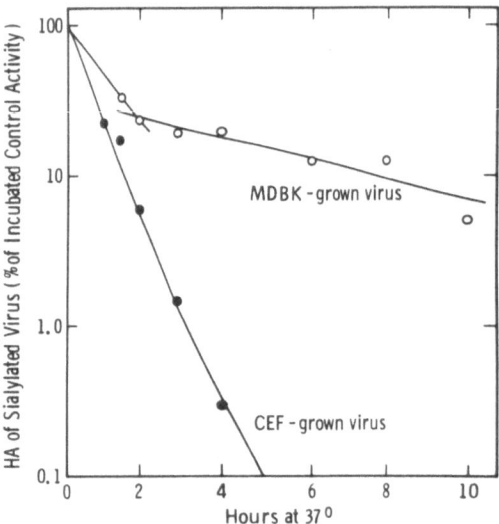

Figure 1

Inactivation of the hemagglutinating activity of influenza virus by sialylation of the virion hemagglutinin. Purified virions of the WSN strain of influenza obtained from MDBK cells or CEF were used. 25,000 HAU were incubated in 0.4 ml of 0.1 M phosphate buffer, pH 6.9 with 1.5 mg of sialyltransferase in the presence and absence of 0.002 μmoles of CMP-sialic acid. At the intervals indicated, aliquots were removed and hemagglutinating activity (HA) was measured using chick erythrocytes (0.5% in phosphate buffered saline). Virions incubated in the absence of CMP-sialic acid lost no hemagglutinating activity.

Kinetic studies revealed that destruction of hemagglutinating activity occurred at a faster rate than did enhancement of infectivity and that a diphasic enhancement response was always obtained, with maximum infectivity being observed after two to four hours of incubation (Schulze, 1975a). Thus, various factors including the state of the virions, the extent of sialylation, and the host used for infectivity measurements appeared to be critical in determining whether enhancement would be observed. Recently we have observed that the source of virus to be sialylated is also of importance. In Figures 1 and 2, virions from two sources, CEF and MDBK cells, are compared. After four hours of sialylation, less than 0.5% of the initial hemagglutinating activity remains with CEF-grown virus; with MDBK-grown virus, 5% of the initial activity still remains after 10 hours of sialylation. In keeping with these observations, we have found that under comparable incubation conditions some 5 to 10 times as much sialic acid is attached to CEF-grown as to MDBK-grown virus. This slower rate of sialylation may also be responsible for the lack of enhancement observed with MDBK-grown virus (Figure 2). Whereas a tenfold increase in the plaque titer of CEF-grown virus was observed after 2 hours of incubation, the maximum increase observed with MDBK-grown virus was less than twofold. Thus, the rate of extent of sialylation and hence the amount of enhancement is determined in part by the composition of the oligosaccharides put onto the hemagglutinin by host cell glycosyltransferases.

Binding of Virions to Erythrocytes and Host Cells

The most straightforward explanation for increasing the infectivity of a virus preparation while destroying its hemagglutinating activity would be that binding to erythrocytes was decreased. Although the complexity of the infectivity enhancement just described argues against such a simple mechanism, we considered binding data to be essential to further interpretation of our findings. Accordingly, we have prepared virus heavily labelled with ^{32}P and have studied its ability to bind to erythrocytes as well as to CEF and MDBK cells. Purified virus obtained from both CEF and MDBK cells has been studied as has neuraminidase-free virus obtained by mild trypsinization.

Virions were sialylated until 10% or less of the hemagglutinating activity remained. They were then reisolated from the reaction mixture by centrifugation and resuspended in appropriate buffers. Unsialylated (control) virions incubated with the enzyme in the absence of CMP-sialic acid were handled in the same way. All of the ^{32}P originally incorporated into virions remained associated with the particles through this treatment. These virus preparations were added to erythrocytes or to host cells at ratios similar to those used to measure hemagglutination and infectivity.

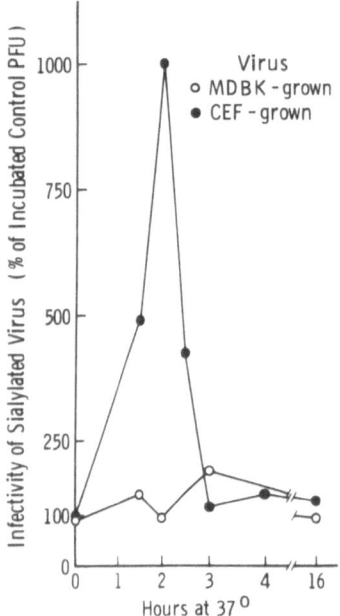

Figure 2

Effect of sialylation on the infectivity of influenza virus. Sialylation was carried out as described for Figure 1. Infectivity was measured as described by Noronha-Blob and Schulze (1976). Incubated controls retained 60% of their initial activity at 2 hours and 12% at 16 hours.

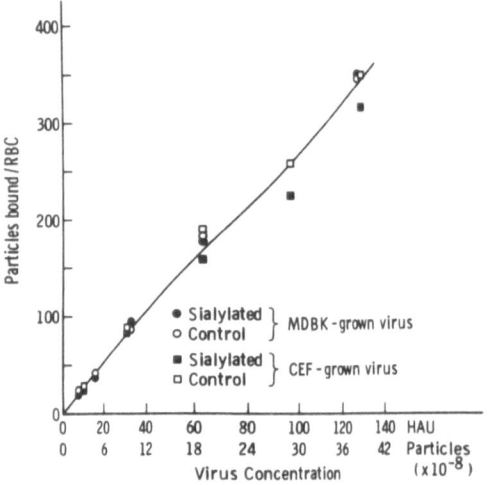

Figure 3

Binding of virions to erythrocytes under conditions of receptor excess. Purified ^{32}P-labelled virions (10,000 HAU) with a specific activity of 10 to 20 ^{32}P cpm/IIAU were incubated at

37° in 0.2 ml of 0.1 M phosphate buffer, pH 6.9, containing 0.002 μmoles (0.4 μCi) CMP-^{14}C-sialic acid and 0.74 mg of sialyltransferase. Controls consisted of identical reaction mixture without CMP-sialic acid. CEF-grown virus was incubated for 4 hours and MDBK-grown virus for 16 hours at which time the residual hemagglutinating activities were 5% or less of the initial values. Both sialylated and control virions were recovered from the reaction mixture by sedimentation through a 30% sucrose cushion by centrifugation at 140,000 x g for 1 hour. The pelleted virus was resuspended in STE (0.05 M Tris, pH 7.5, 0.1 M NaCl and 10^{-3} M EDTA). The specific activity (^{32}P cpm/HAU) were again determined for the incubated control and was found to be unchanged by incubation. Varying concentrations of sialylated and control virus were mixed with 10^{7} erythrocytes in a final volume 0.5 ml of phosphate buffered saline. After 1 hour at room temperature, the erythrocytes were pelleted, (1000 x g for 10 minutes) washed thrice in phosphate buffered saline and repelleted. Pellets were solubilized by addition of 1 ml of 0.1 N NaOH; the ^{32}P associated with the pellets, the supernatant fractions, and the washes were determined to ensure complete recovery of virus. Particles bound/RBC was then calculated from the amount of ^{32}P associated with the pellet and the specific activity of the virus preparation. One HAU was taken to be 3 x 10^{7} virions. The HAU values on the ordinate refer to activities prior to sialylation.

Figure 3 presents data representative of that obtained when binding to approximately 10^{7} erythrocytes was measured. The amount of virus bound was linearly related to the added virus, indicating that an excess of binding sites was available. At the highest concentration of virus used in this experiment, some 300 virions were bound per cell.

Under these conditions, sialylated virions from both host cells were bound to erythrocytes to the same extent as were incubated control virions. Thus, when receptor sites are not limiting, 85% or more of the added virus can bind to erythrocytes.

Figure 4 presents data obtained from similar experiments in which binding to monolayers of MDBK cells was measured. Again the amount of binding was linear with virus addition and no differences between sialylated and control viruses were observed. However, in these experiments the amount of virus per cell depended on the source of the virus. Although some variation in binding was observed from experiment to experiment, approximately twice as many MDBK cell-grown virions were bound per cell as were CEF-grown virions.

The maximum amount of virus which could be bound to MDBK cells was approximately 60%, whereas 85 to 90% was bound to erythrocytes. Sequential treatment of virus suspensions with MDBK cells and erythrocytes showed that those virions which were not taken up by MDBK cells were capable of binding to erythrocytes (Figure 5). Thus, about 25% of the particles which bind to erythrocytes appear to have a low affinity for MDBK cells so that, even under conditions of large receptor excess, they fail to bind.

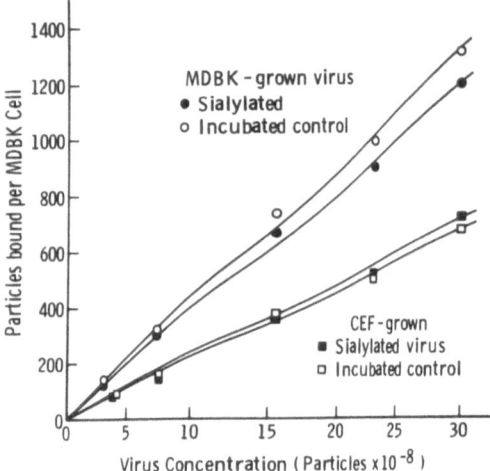

Figure 4

Binding of virions to host cells under conditions of receptor excess. Experiments were carried out as described for **Figure 3** except that binding to monolayers consisting of 6 x 10^5 cells was measured. Monolayers were washed with buffered isotonic saline (SBS; Mandel, 1958) and incubated at room temperature for 1 hour, with various concentrations of virus in 50 μl of GSBS (SBS containing 1% gelatin). During the incubation period the plates were rocked at 15 minute intervals. Unbound virus was removed from the monolayers, the monolayers were washed thrice and then solubilized by addition of 0.1 N NaOH. The amount of virus bound per cell was determined as described above.

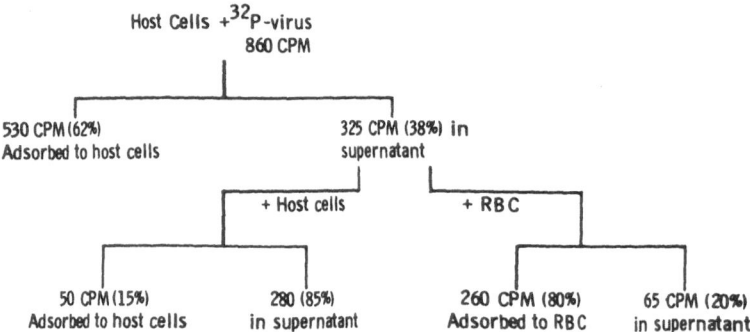

Figure 5

A comparison of binding of influenza virus to host cells and to erythrocytes. The amount of ^{32}P-labelled virus bound to each type of cell was determined as described for Figures 3 and 4.

Trypsinized virus gave identical results to those presented in Figures 3 and 4, indicating that neither removal of neuraminidase and the cleavage of HA to HA_1 and HA_2 nor subsequent sialylation of such trypsin-treated virus altered binding under conditions of receptor excess.

The experiments just described clearly show that the changes in biological activities induced by sialylation did not reflect decreased binding to erythrocytes or increased binding to MDBK cells. They also suggested that a vastly different receptor-virus ratio would be necessary in order to detect small differences in the affinity, heterogeneity, and number of virus receptors on host cells and on erythrocytes. For example, since under conditions of receptor excess, 60% of the control virus could bind to MDBK cells, changes in binding of comparable magnitude to the increases in infectivity (i.e., 10-fold increases) could not be expected. Accordingly, conditions were sought under which the amount of virus bound would be determined by limiting receptors rather than by limiting virus. Binding studies were carried out using 10^5 erythrocytes instead of 10^7 and virus concentrations were increased 100-fold. As shown in Figure 6, at a virus to cell ratio of approximately 6×10^6, erythrocytes are nearly saturated with virus particles. Under these conditions, 5×10^5 particles can be adsorbed per erythrocyte. This value greatly exceeds those of 5×10^3 to 10×10^3 virions per cell previously obtained from electron microscopic counts of the number of virus particles per unit of erythrocyte membrane (Dawson and Elford, 1949) or from measuring the residual hemagglutinating activity of virus suspensions after treatment with erythrocytes (Bateman et al., 1955). Since neither of these methods provided both optimum conditions for binding and a large excess of virus particles, the number of receptors per cell calculated from the data may be falsely low. However, our binding data obtained at saturation also does not represent the number of receptor sites per cell since the number of particles adsorbed appears to be in excess of that which can be accommodated on the surface of the cell. The surface area of lysed chicken erythrocyte membranes had been determined to be about 180 square microns (Dawson and Elford, 1949), and can therefore accommodate no more than about 25,000 spherical virions 1000 Å in diameter. Under saturating conditions, virions appear to aggregate onto the surface of the erythrocytes so that the number of virus binding sites on the cell itself cannot be determined from the number of particles bound.

Comparable binding studies using host cells were carried out in plates with small wells which contained monolayers consisting of 5×10^5 CEF or 6×10^5 MDBK cells. As shown in Figure 7a, approximately 7×10^{10} virions were required to saturate the CEF monolayers; at that concentration and above,

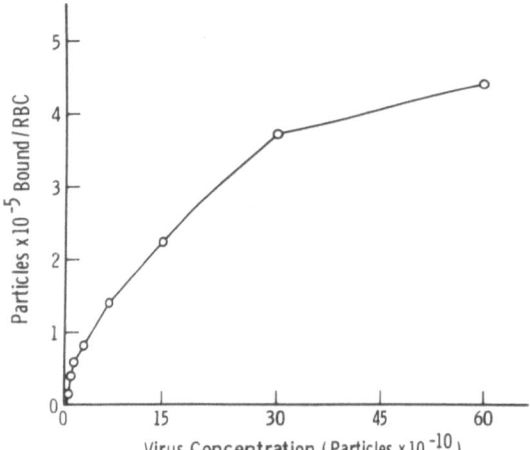

Figure 6

Saturation of erythrocytes with influenza virions. **Binding of purified ^{32}P-labelled virus to erythrocytes was measured as described in Figure 3 except that the cell concentration was reduced to 10^5 cells per assay.**

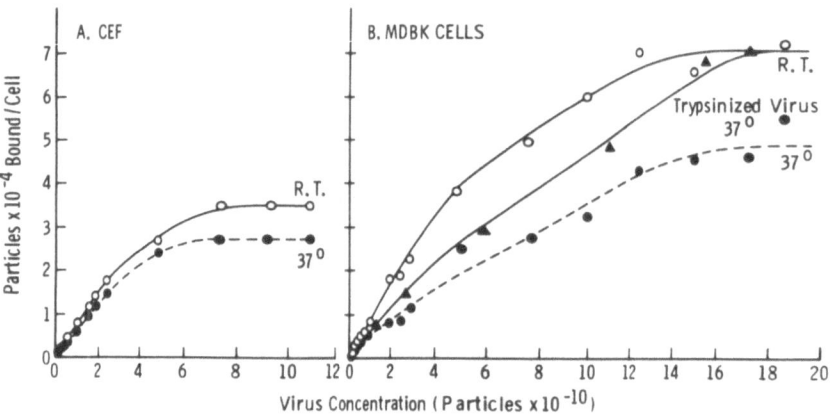

Figure 7

A comparison of the influenza virus binding capacity to CEF and MDBK cells. Experiments using purified ^{32}P-labelled virus were carried out as described for Figure 4, except that CEF monolayers contained 5×10^5 cells.

2.7×10^4 particles were bound per cell at 37°, whereas 3.5×10^4 were bound at room temperature. Approximately twice as much virus is required to saturate MDBK cells (**Figure 7b**); under these conditions 5×10^4 virions are bound per MDBK cell at 37° and 7×10^4 at room temperature. The effect on binding of trypsinizing the virus is also shown in **Figure 7b**. Virions devoid of neuraminidase show increased binding at 37° as compared with intact virus. At room temperature binding like that shown for intact virus was observed. The results suggest that at 37° the viral neuraminidase on intact virions reduces the fraction of virus bound at all virus concentrations by reducing the total number of binding sites on MDBK cells.

Having determined the maximum number of virions which can bind to MDBK cells, binding of sialylated and incubated control virions could be compared under conditions approaching saturation. As shown in Figure 8, no differences in binding were detected at virus concentrations up to 12×10^{10} particles per assay. Assuming that each virion bound at saturation represents a receptor site, Figures 4 and 8 together present data obtained at virus to receptor ratios ranging from 10^{-2} to 5.

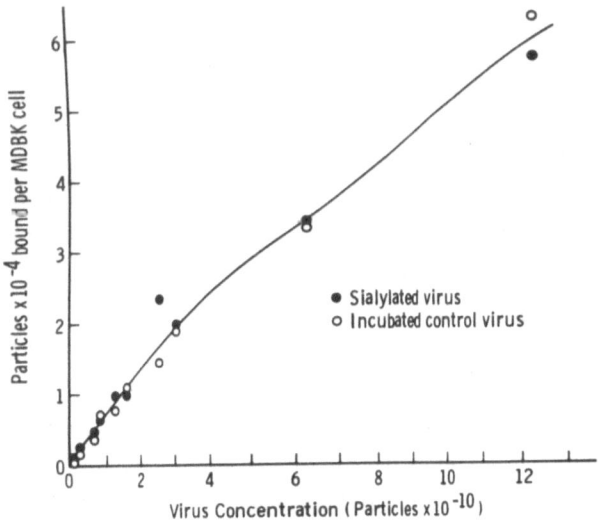

Figure 8

Binding of virions to host cells under conditions of limiting receptor concentrations. Experiments were carried out as described for Figure 4.

Experiments aimed at evaluating the contribution of 'nonspecific' binding to data obtained with both erythrocytes and host cells are in progress. Since hemagglutination can be reversed and virions can be eluted by the action of viral neuraminidase on erythrocyte glycoproteins, nonspecific binding can be defined as that which is observed at neutral pH after sialic acid residues are removed from erythrocytes. However, there is no direct evidence that infection is initiated only by the attachment of virions to sialylated receptors on host cells. For these cells specific binding should therefore be defined as that which can lead to infection, rather than as that involving sialic acid containing receptors. Using this definition, no clear-cut experimental approach determining specific binding is available. Until more information concerning the receptor activity of host cell membrane fractions is available, the only criteria at hand are those applied to other receptor-ligand interactions (see Cuatrecasas, 1975). These include saturability and high affinity, both of which can be evaluated in this system.

Except for the possibility that changes in specific binding are masked by non-specific interactions, these data indicate that changes in binding *per se* are not responsible for the enhancement of infectivity brought about by sialylation. Thus the enhancement may be due (a) to the formation of infectious aggregates from defective particles (Hirst and Pons, 1973), (b) to an increased ability of sialylated virus to penetrate host cells and to initiate infections, or (c) to a combination of these two mechanisms.

Since covalent attachment of sialic acid to some but not all of the galactoses on the hemagglutinin might be expected to lead to aggregation, we have examined the sedimentation properties of both sialylated virus and virus which was incubated with sialyltransferase alone (incubated control virus). As shown in Figure 9, both preparations of virus are aggregated. Based on the position of the aggregated particles relative to that of the monodisperse virus, each aggregate contains 8 or more virions.

Since the incubated control virus preparations contained approximately 10^4 PFU (on MDBK cells) per HAU, aggregates of 8 particles would be highly unlikely to contain more than one infectious virion. Thus, loss of infectivity due to aggregate formation was not expected and was not observed. However, if aggregation alone were able to enhance infectivity by forming infectious units from defective particles, non-sialylated aggregates should be as infectious as are sialylated ones. Since this is not the case, sialylation must either form more stable aggregates or facilitate penetration of the cell membrane by the aggregates.

Enhancement of Infectivity by Hemagglutination Inhibitors

Another approach to the study of influenza virus receptors is the use of soluble sialoglycoproteins which are capable of binding to virions and inhibiting hemagglutination. These substances are found in the serum of most species (see

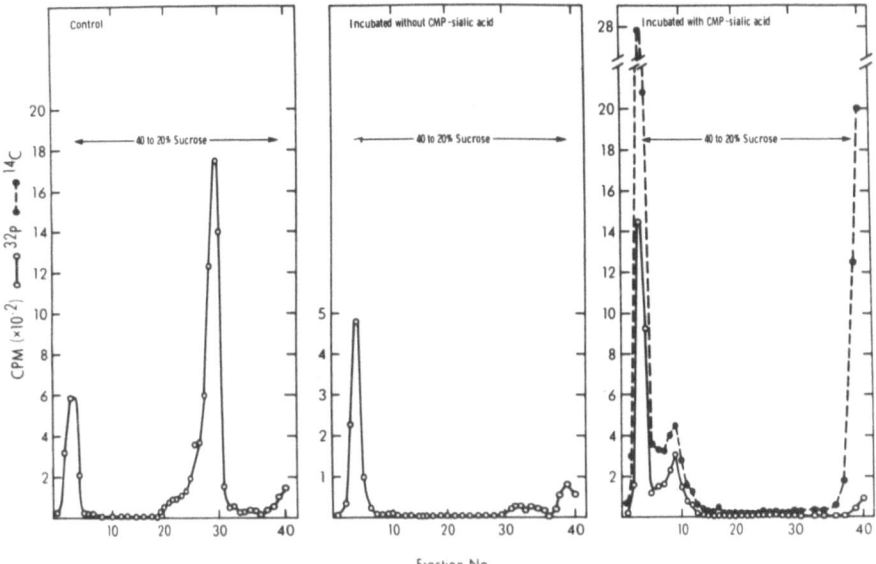

Figure 9

Sedimentation profiles of sialylated and control virus. Purified ^{32}P-labelled CEF-grown
virions were incubated for 2 hours with and without CMP-sialic acid as described for Figure
3. The infectivity of the sialylated virus was 5 times that of the incubated control virus.
Virions recovered from the reaction mixtures by sedimentation to equilibrium in a sucrose
gradient were concentrated by centrifugation at 140,000 x g for 70 minutes, resuspended in
phosphate buffered saline and overlaid onto a 10 ml 20% to 40% sucrose gradient on top a
1 ml cushion of 60% sucrose. Purified virions were applied to a third gradient. After centrifugation for 1 hour at 25,000 rpm in a SW41 rotor, fractions were collected from the bottom
of the tube.

Krizanova and Rathova, 1969). While some also neutralize infectivity, others
fail to do so, and it has been proposed that the viral neuraminidase fosters infection *in vivo* by destroying these inhibitors which would otherwise bind to the
viral hemagglutinin and prevent adsorption of the virus to cells which support
virus growth.

Since fully infectious virions devoid of neuraminidase activity can be obtained
by trypsinization (Schulze, 1970), this proposal could be tested directly.
Virions without neuraminidase activity should not be released from these glycoproteins and should be inactivated by glycoprotein concentrations which
prevent hemagglutination. In order to test this hypothesis, fetuin, a well characterized glycoprotein known to be an inhibitor of hemagglutination, was used.

Table 1

Effect of Fetuin on the Hemagglutinating Activity and Infectivity of Influenza
Virus

Virus	Fetuin Conc. (mg/ml)	HAU/ml	PFU/ml ($\times 10^{-6}$)	PFU/HA
Intact	-	400	2.8	7.0×10^3
	2.1	20	16	8.0×10^5
Trypsin-treated	-	400	4.9	1.2×10^4
	2.1	10	20	2.0×10^6

As shown in Table 1, whereas the hemagglutinating activity of intact and trypsinized virus was destroyed by fetuin, the infectivity of both preparations was
increased. Similar results were obtained when infectivity was measured on CEF
except that the enhancement was approximately one half that observed on
MDBK monolayers. Submaxillary mucin also gave similar results. Clearly,
release of virions from glycoproteins by viral neuraminidase is not a prerequisite
for establishing infection.

Table 2

Effects of Fetuin and Desialofetuin on Influenza Virus

Virus	conc. HAU/ml	Treatment (5 μg/HA)	% of Control Activity	
			HA	Infectivity
Intact	70	Fetuin	5	600
		Desialofetuin	100	109
Trypsin-treated	70	Fetuin	4	1100
		Desialofetuin	100	282

That sialic acid residues are implicated in enhancement as well as in inhibition
is shown in Table 2. Removal of sialic acid residues from the fetuin by mild acid
hydrolysis eliminated both effects. Mild oxidation and reduction of fetuin (a
treatment which shortens the polyhydroxyl side chain of sialic acid residues on
glycoproteins without inducing large changes in the remainder of the molecules
(Van Lenten and Ashwell, 1972)) also eliminated both effects. Fetuin modified

in this manner has been previously shown to be inactive as an inhibitor of hem-agglutination and to be a poor substrate for the viral neuraminidase (Suttajit and Winzler, 1971; Schulze, 1975).

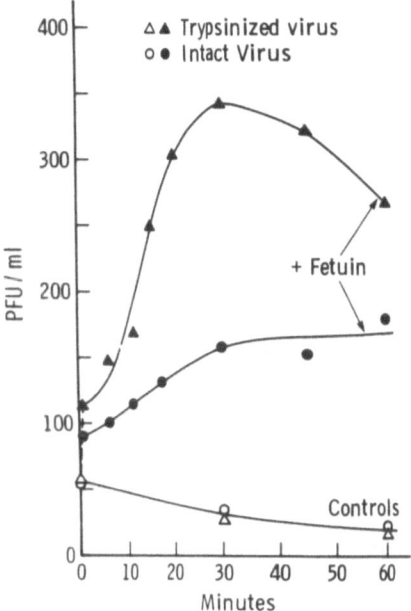

Figure 10

Kinetics of enhancement of infectivity of influenza virus by fetuin. 420 HAU of purified intact or trypsinized influenza virus was incubated with 2.1 mg of fetuin in a final volume of 3.5 ml of phosphate buffered saline. Controls consisted of virus in buffer alone. At intervals after the addition of fetuin, the infectivity of the preparations was measured on MDBK cells. Values on the abscissa are plaques per ml at a 10^{-4} dilution of the reaction mixture.

Kinetic analysis showed that the loss of hemagglutinating activity occurred almost immediately after addition of fetuin (not shown), whereas at a concentration of 5µg/HAU about 30 minutes were required for maximum enhancement of infectivity (Figure 10). These experiments were carried out at 50 to 200 HAU per ml, because greater enhancement was obtained at low virus concentrations. Under these conditions, maximum enhancement was obtained at a concentration of 3 to 5 µg of fetuin per HAU (Figure 11). This amount of fetuin provides in the order of 10^6 molecules per virion, an inhibitor to virus ratio which would be expected to saturate all hemagglutinin spikes.

Sedimentation profiles of influenza virions treated with fetuin or with desialo-fetuin at 5 µg/HAU are presented in Figure 12. Aggregation occurs only when

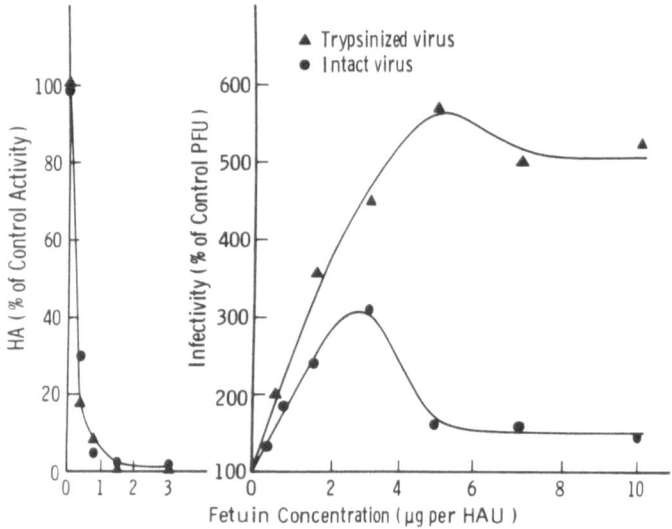

Figure 11

Effect of fetuin concentration on extent of enhancement. 60 HAU of purified intact or trypsinized virus was incubated in 0.5 ml of phosphate buffered saline containing varying concentrations of fetuin for 1 hour at 37°. Virus in phosphate buffer saline served as controls.
Infectivity and hemagglutinating activity was measured as described in Figures 1 and 2.

Table 3

Effect of Fetuin on Hemagglutination and on Binding of Virus to Erythrocytes

Virus HAU/ml	Fetuin (μg/HA)	Percentage of Control Activity HA	Binding
Intact 40,000	-	100	100
	0.01	0.5	98
Trypsinized 80,000	-	100	100
	0.01	2.0	93

the fetuin is sialylated. The modified fetuin containing the 7-carbon analogues
of sialic acid described above also failed to aggregate the virus particles (not
shown). Thus, as has been observed with sialylated virions, increases in infectivity are observed along with the formation of viral aggregates.

As was observed with the sialylated virions, inhibition of hemagglutinating
activity by fetuin was not due to the elimination of binding of virus to erythro-

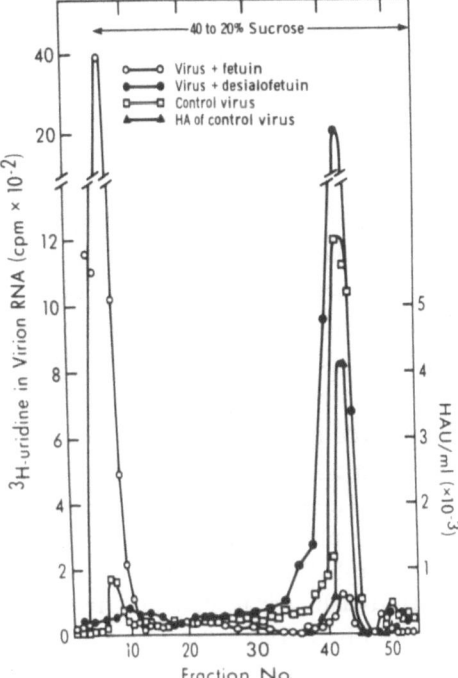

Figure 12

Sedimentation velocity study of virion after treatment with fetuin and desialyfetuin. 2000 HAU of ^{3}H-uridine-labelled virus was incubated with fetuin or desialofetuin at a concentration of 5 μg/HAU as described for Figure 11. Control virus was incubated in phosphate buffered saline alone. 0.2 ml of each sample was put onto sucrose gradients and centrifuged as described for Figure 9. The uridine counts represent the total TCA precipitable counts in each sample.

cytes. Table 3 shows that concentrations of fetuin which reduced hemagglutinating activity to 2% or less failed to inhibit binding. Comparable results have been obtained in preliminary experiments with host cells; in this case, however, concentrations of fetuin which stimulate infectivity appear to slightly reduce binding.

The experiments indicate that virions aggregated by fetuin can be taken up by MDBK cells and that such aggregates are more infectious than is monodisperse virus.

Conclusions

The series of experiments described here indicates that the infectivity of influenza virions does not depend on their hemagglutinin spikes being free of either

covalently linked sialic acid residues or of glycoproteins, whereas their hemagglutinating activity does. These apparently divergent effects are easily recon-
ciled now that we have found that loss of hemagglutinating activity does not
mean that the virus is no longer binding to erythrocytes. Thus, under the conditions used to monitor biological activities as well as under conditions of
limiting receptor concentration, sialylation of the virus has little effect on its
ability to bind to either host cells or erythrocytes. With both types of cells, the
change in biological activity must therefore involve either changes in binding
properties which cannot be detected by the methods used, or secondary effects
controlled in part by the properties of the cell. Our results with sialylated glycoproteins suggest a similar mechanism. Again, these glycoproteins must either
change the manner in which virions bind to cells or induce changes which follow binding. The degree of enhancement observed depends on the source of the
virus, trypsin treatment of the virus prior to addition of sialic acid or fetuin, and
the host cell on which infectivity is monitored. Therefore, it is unlikely that
complementation following aggregation of incomplete particles analogous to
that of Hirst and Pons (1973) is totally responsible for the observed increases
in plaque forming units. Rather, it appears that sialic acid residues on the virions
change their interactions with the host cell membranes in a manner which facili-
tates uptake of virions be they monodisperse or aggregated.

Independent of the mechanism of enhancement, it is clear that virus preparations which lack hemagglutinating activity may show enhanced infectivity. These
observations, along with those which show that trypsin-induced changes in the
hemagglutinin can alter the infectivity of virus preparations without changing
their hemagglutinating activity (Lazarowitz and Choppin, 1975; Klenk *et al.*,
1976), indicate that the ratio of these two activities tells one little about the
genetic competence of virus preparations.

Our results also prompt one to consider whether sialylated virions ever exist in
nature. Even when sialylated virus is aggregated it is at least as infectious as is
monodisperse unsialylated virus. Consequently, if the process which keeps
virions free of sialic acid were to function poorly under some conditions, virus
released from the cell would be expected to be infectious, even if aggregated, so
long as the aggregates could re-enter cells. If such virions do exist in nature,
they might be expected to be altered in virulence since sialic acid residues on
soluble glycoproteins (Morell *et al.*, 1971) as well as on hepatitis B surface antigens (Neurath *et al.*, 1975) alter the interactions of these molecules with cell
receptors.

Another consideration which our results bring to mind is whether some soluble
glycoproteins foster infection *in vivo*. Since the infectivity of neuraminidase-

free virus can be enhanced rather than inhibited, virions can apparently bind to cells while still bound to some glycoproteins. Are such virions presented to host cells in a fashion that promotes complementation and recombination between defective particles? Do the secretions of the respiratory mucosa therefore make it possible for defective particles to operate more, instead of less, efficiently? Such questions can presumably be answered by careful analysis of the inter-action of influenza virions with host cell receptors.

Acknowledgements

We wish to thank Miss Mieko Osuga for excellent technical assistance. Supported by Grant AI-10097 from the National Institute of Allergy and Infectious Disease, U.S. Public Health Service.

REFERENCES

BARTHOLOMEW, B. A. and JOURDIAN, G. W. (1966) in 'Methods in Enzymology' (Neufeld, E. F. and Ginsburg, V., eds.) Vol. 8, pp. 368, Academic Press, New York.
BATEMAN, J. B., DAVIS, M. S. and McCAFFREY, P. A. (1955) Am. J. Hyg. 62, 349-354.
CUATRECASAS, P. (1976) in 'Advances in Cyclic Nucleotide Research' (Drummond, G. I. and Robinson, G. A., eds.) Vol. 5, pp. 79, Raven Press, New York.
DAWSON, I. M. and ELFORD, W. J. (1949) J. Gen. Microbiol. 3, 298-311.
EYLAR, E. H., MADOFF, M. A., BRODY, O. V. and ONCLEY, J. L. (1972) J. Biol. Chem. 237, 1992-2000.
GLICK, M. C., COMSTOCK, C. and WARREN, L. (1970) Biochem. Biophys. Acta. 219, 290-300.
HUGHES, R. C. (1973) Prog. Biophys. Mol. Biol. 26, 189-268.
HIRST, G. K. and PONS, M. W. (1973) Virology 56, 620-631.
KLENK, H-D. and CHOPPIN, P. W. (1970) Proc. Nat. Acad. Sci. USA. 66, 57-64.
KLENK, H-D., CALIGUIRI, L. A. and CHOPPIN, P. W. (1970a) Virology 42, 473-481.
KLENK, H-D., COMPANS, R. W. and CHOPPIN, P. W. (1970b) Virology 42, 1158-1162.
KLENK, H-D., ROTT, R., ORLICH, M. and BLÖDORN, J. (1975) Virology 68, 426-439.
KRIZANOVA, O. and RATHOVA, V. (1969) Curr. Top-Microbiol. Immunol. 47, 125-151.
LAKSHMI, M. V., DER, C-L. and SCHULZE, I. T. (1976) Fed. Proc. 35, 1432.
LAKSHMI, M. V. and SCHULZE, I. T. (1977) Manuscript in preparation.
LAVER, W. G. (1971) Virology 45, 275-288.
LAZAROWITZ, S. G., COMPANS, R. W. and CHOPPIN, P. W. (1971) Virology 46, 830-843.
LAZAROWITZ, S. G. and CHOPPIN, P. W. (1975) Virology 68, 440-454.
MADIN, S. H. and DARBY, N. B. Jr. (1958) Proc. Soc. Exp. Biol. Med. 98, 574-580.
MANDEL, B. (1958) Virology 6, 424-447.
MORELL, A. G., GREGORIADIS, G., SCHEINBERG, H. I., HICKMAN, J. and ASHWELL, G. (1971) J. Biol. Chem. 246, 1461-1467.
NEURATH, A. R., HASHIMOTO, N. and PRINCE, A. M. (1975) J. Gen. Virol. 27, 81-91.
NORONHA-BLOB, L. and SCHULZE, I. T. (1976) Virology 69, 314-322.
SCHULZE, I. T. (1970) Virology 42, 890-904.
SCHULZE, I. T. (1972) Virology 47, 181-196.

SCHULZE, I. T. (1973) Advan. Virus Res. *18*, 1-55.

SCHULZE, I. T. (1975) in 'Influenza Viruses and Influenza' (Kilbourne, E. D., ed.) pp. 53, Academic Press, New York.

SCHULZE, I. T. (1975a) in 'Negative Strand Viruses' (Barry, R. D. and Mahy, B. W. J., eds.) Vol. 1, pp. 161, Academic Press, New York.

SUTTAJIT, M. and WINZLER, R. J. (1971) J. Biol. Chem. *246*, 3398-3404.

VAN LENTEN. L. and ASHWELL, G. (1971) J. Biol. Chem. *246*, 1889-1894.

WINZLER, R. J. (1969). In 'Red Cell Membrane, Structure and Function' (Jamieson, G. A. and Greenwald, T. J., eds.), p. 157. Lippincott, Philadelphia, Pennsylvania.

ELECTRON MICROSCOPY OF ANTIBODIES BOUND TO ISOLATED INFLUENZA HEMAGGLUTININ

Nicholas G. Wrigley and W. Graeme Laver

Influenza virus particles possess two antigens on their surface, hemagglutinin and neuraminidase. Antibody directed against the former neutralizes virus infectivity, yet continual antigenic variation renders this neutralization ineffective and allows recurrent epidemics of influenza in man.

Hemagglutinin is a rod-shaped glycoprotein of about 220,000 molecular weight and one end (the 'proximal' end) possesses hydrophobic regions which are associated with the lipid envelope of the intact virus (Schulze, 1973). Complete hemagglutinin may be extracted by disruption of the virus with sodium dodecyl sulfate; proteolytic digestion of the virus with Bromelain gives an incomplete hemagglutinin which has lost its hydrophobic portions. This paper describes the binding of antibodies to both complete and incomplete forms. Two kinds of antibody were used, one being specific to the Hong Kong/68 hemagglutinin against which it was raised, and the other having common reactivity with the related Memphis/102/72 strain.

Materials and Methods

Viruses

A recombinant influenza virus possessing the hemagglutinin subunits of Hong Kong influenza and A/BEL neuraminidase (A/Hong Kong/68H-A/BEL/42N; H3N1) was the source of the hemagglutinin subunits. Hemagglutinin from this particular strain is unusually resistant to the action of SDS, and so is more likely to survive intact after disruption of virus. The other virus used in the preparation of antisera was A/Memphis/102/72 (H3N2). The viruses were grown in the allantoic sac of 11-day old chicken embryos and purified by adsorption on and elution from chicken erythrocytes followed by differential centrifugation and sedimentation through a sucrose gradient as described by Laver (1969).

Isolation of Hemagglutinin

'Complete' hemagglutinin molecules were isolated by electrophoresis on cellulose acetate strips after disruption of the virus particles with SDS as described previously (Laver and Valentine, 1969; Laver and Webster, 1973). Partially degraded (incomplete) hemagglutinin molecules were isolated by proteolytic digestion of the virus particles with Bromelain (Sigma) and purified by sucrose density gradient (Brand and Skehel, 1972). Hemagglutinin titrations were done using chicken erythrocytes, and the incomplete molecules, having lost the ability to attach to red cells after Bromelain digestion, were detected by double immunodiffusion tests in agar.

Preparation of Purified Immunoglobulin G Antibody Molecules

Antibodies to the specific and the common antigenic determinants of the hemagglutinin molecules of Hong Kong influenza virus were prepared in a way similar to that described by Laver et al. (1974). Hyperimmune rabbit antiserum to the isolated hemagglutinin molecules of SDS-disrupted A/Hong Kong/68 influenza virus was prepared. This antiserum was then absorbed with purified A/Memphis/102/72 virus until all of the common antibody was removed. This antibody was then dissociated from the virus particles at pH 3.0 as described, except that the 0.1 M glycine-HCl buffer used for the dissociation did not contain any added protein (Laver et al., 1974). It is probable that the most avid antibody was lost, but most of the antibody activity was recovered and showed the same cross-reactions as before absorption-dissociation. The serum remaining after removal of the common antibody was then absorbed with purified particles of A/Hong Kong/68 virus and the specific antibody dissociated from the virus in the same way. The common and specific IgG antibody molecules were then purified further by sucrose gradient centrifugation. Samples (0.2 ml) of the dissociated antibodies were layered onto 5 ml sucrose gradients (5% to 20% sucrose in 0.15 M NaCl, 0.01 M sodium phosphate, pH 7.2) and centrifuged at 50,000 revs/min in the SW65 rotor (Beckman Inc.) for 7 h at 20°C. Twenty fractions were collected from a hole in the bottom of the tube and tested for antibody in a microprecipitin test with Hong Kong/68 virus particles. Antibody was present in fractions 10 to 13 which were pooled, dialyzed against phosphate-buffered saline and stored at 4°C after the addition of sodium azide to prevent bacterial growth.

Electron Microscopy

All specimens were examined in a Philips EM 301 electron microscope operated at 80 kV. Specimens were prepared by fist stripping a thin carbon film off mica directly onto a suspension of the molecules to be examined and allowing them to adsorb briefly to the 'virgin' undersurface of the carbon. The concentration of the suspensions was very important, and several dilutions in physiological saline were examined until the observed degree of spreading was obtained, usually around 50 μg/ml. The film was then floated on negative stain (2% aqueous sodium silicotungstate), picked up on a copper grid and air dried. Exposures in the electron microscope were made using techniques to minimize the electron dose and so reduce radiation damage to the specimen.

Preparation of Antigen-Antibody Complexes

The two purified antibody preparations were mixed separately with the two hemagglutinins (complete and incomplete forms). The common anti-hemagglutinin antibody bound to both hemagglutinins, and the specific bound only to the A/HK/68 hemagglutinin.

The relative concentrations of IgG and antigen in any mixture were varied over a wide range to increasing proportions of antibody. The object was to reach such proportions that there were some free IgG molecules remaining after 20 to 30 min at 4°C, indicating saturation of all possible antibody binding sites on the antigen. Unfortunately, this condition was seldom observed in the case of complete antigens because the complexes grew to such large sizes and complexity as to be uninterpretable in the electron microscope. The trends were clear enough, however, especially in incomplete antigen complexes which were much smaller.

Absolute proportions of antigen and antibody were not determined, nor was any systematic attempt made to investigate the preferential occupation of antigenic sites with increasing proportions of antibody. Mixing of common and specific antibody simultaneously with their common antigen was not attempted either.

Results and Discussion

Complexes of the complete Hong Kong/68 hemagglutinin with common and specific antibody are shown in Figures 1 and 2 respectively. These preparations contained concentrations (about 0.01%) of SDS just large enough to prevent too much hydrophobic aggregation of the hemagglutinin molecules, yet low enough to allow satisfactory negative staining. Nevertheless, characteristic 'rosettes' of aggregated hemagglutinin rods were seen (Laver and Valentine, 1969), hydrophobically linked at their proximal ends. In addition, however, there were many instances of rods linked at their distal ends by characteristically Y-shaped IgG molecules. Exactly similar pictures were obtained with both common and specific antibodies.

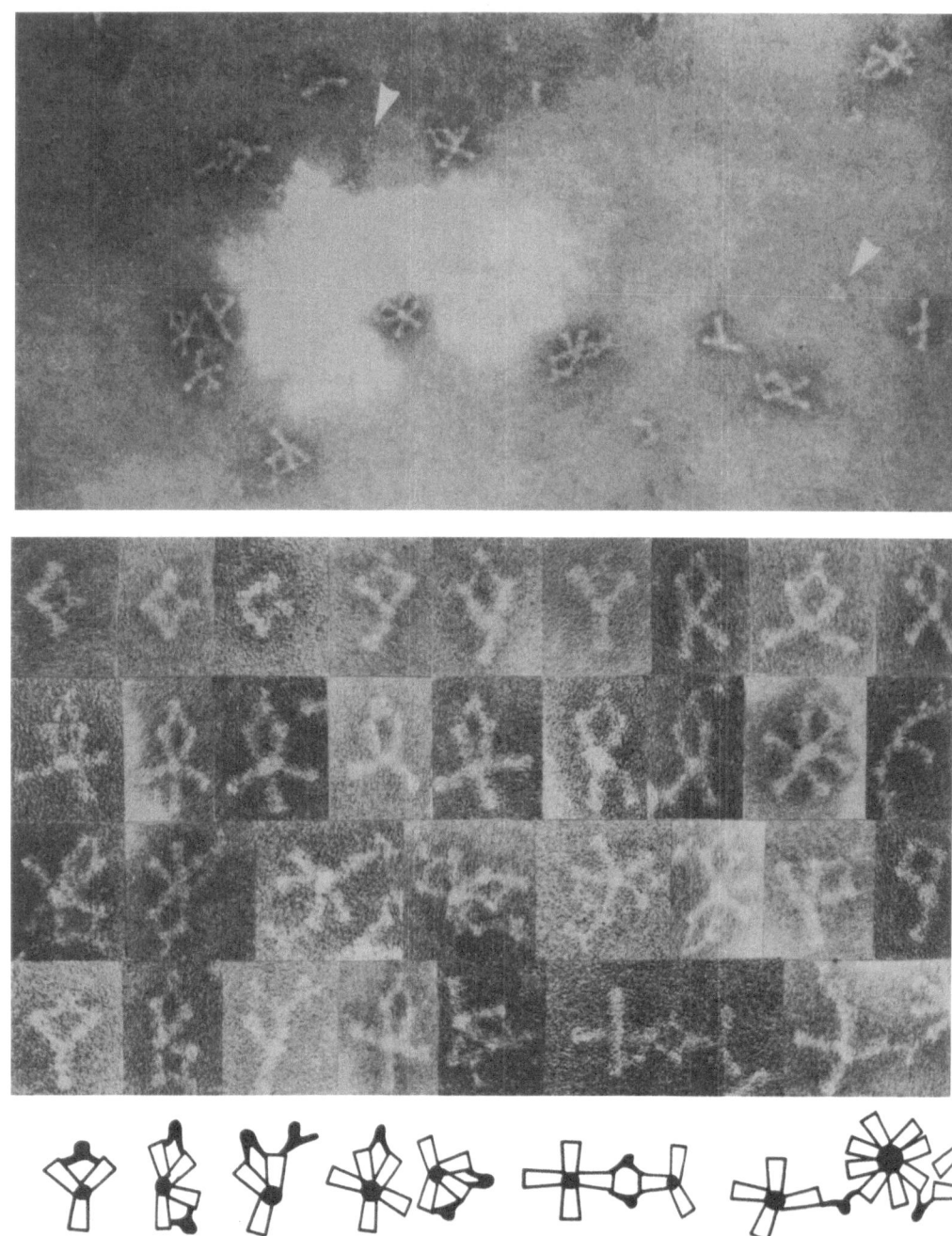

Figure 1

Rosettes of complete hemagglutinin complexed with common IgG antibody.

125

Top: General field at x 200,000, two free IgG molecules arrowed.

Center: Selected complexes from many fields as above, at x 400,000.

Bottom: Sketches of the complexes immediately above. Open rectangles are hemagglutin-
            in rods, with black circles at rosette centers and black IgG molecules bridging
            distal ends.

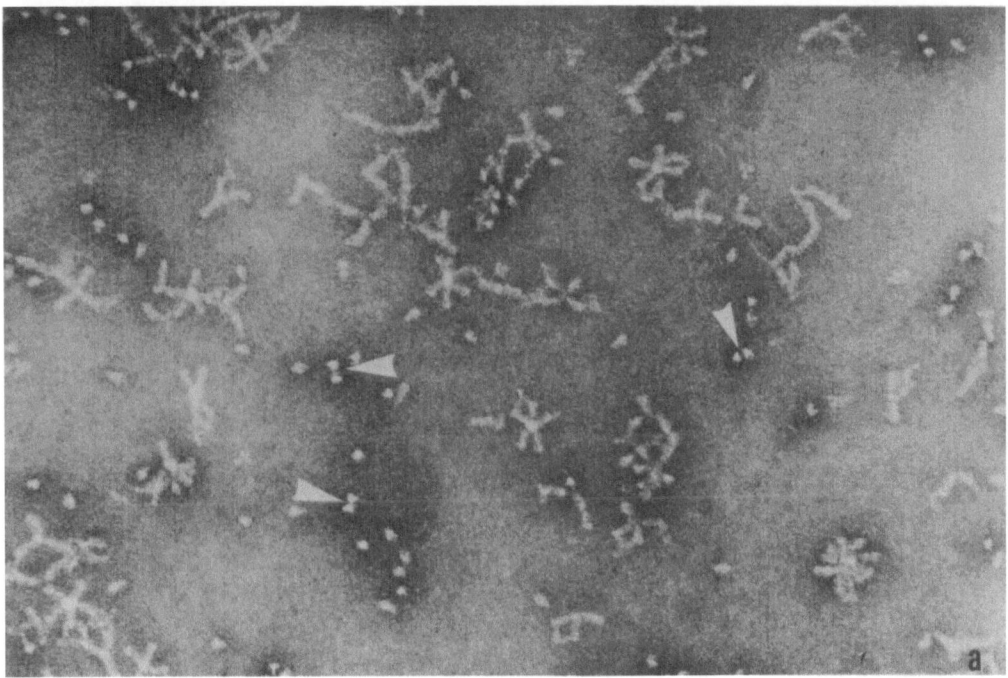

Figure 2a

Rosettes of complete hemagglutinin complexed with specific IgG. General field at x 200,000
some hemagglutinin molecules seen end-on, arrowed.

The binding of common and specific antibodies to the incomplete Hong Kong/
68 hemagglutinin is shown in Figures 3 and 4 respectively. This hemagglutinin,
lacking its hydrophobic 'proximal' end, is slightly shorter than the complete
form and shows no tendency to aggregate into rosettes even in the total absence
of SDS. Nevertheless, after mixing with the antibodies, numerous complexes
were found, ranging from one antigen carrying a single antibody, to long chains
and closed loops of alternating antigen and antibody. As with the complete
hemagglutinin, there was no apparent difference between complexes containing
common or specific antibody.

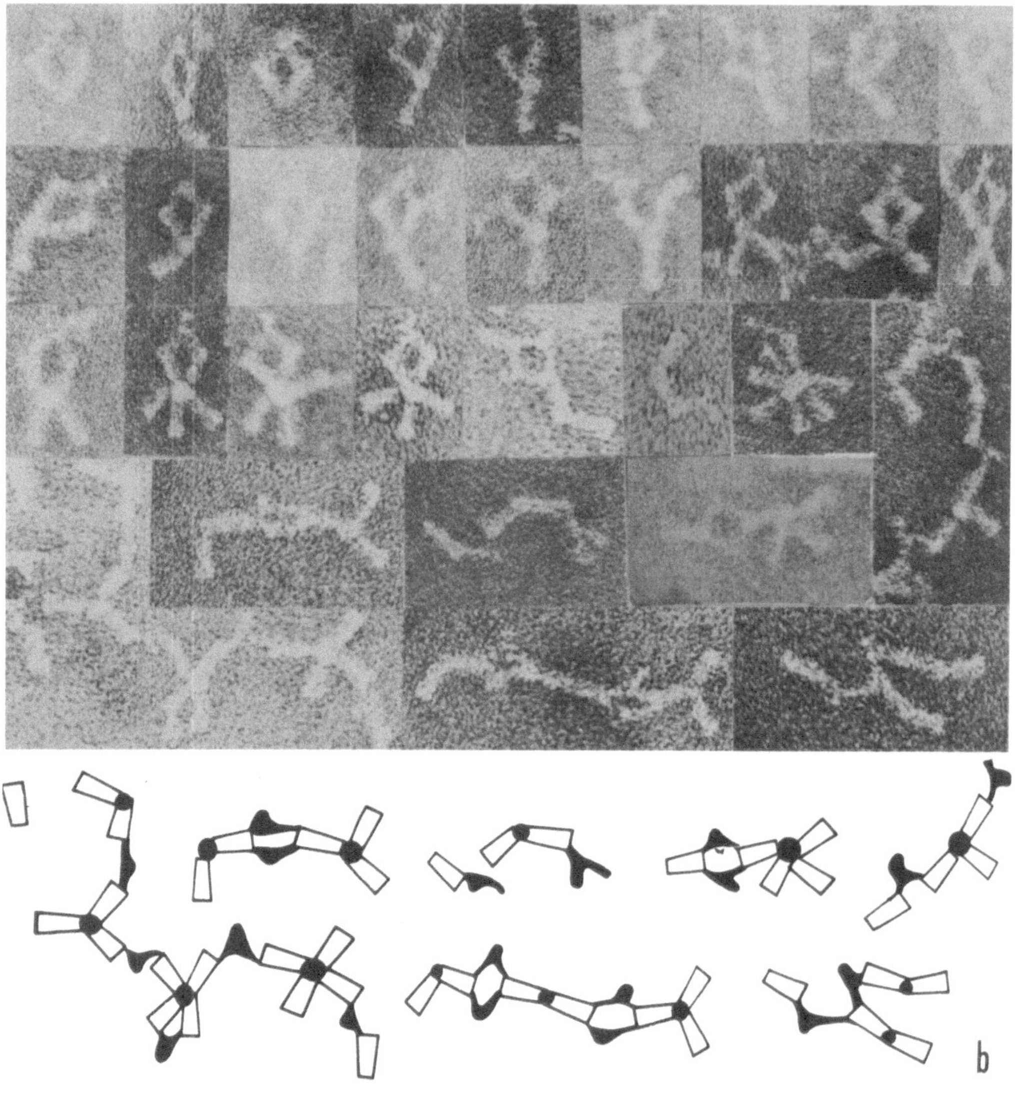

126

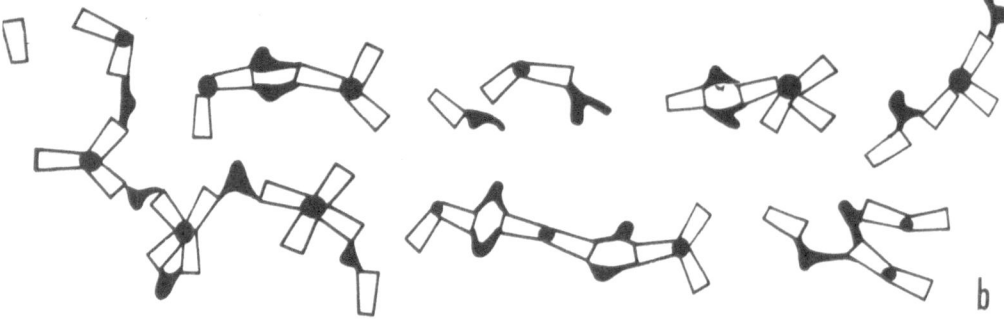

Figure 2b

Rosettes of complete hemagglutinin, complexed with specific IgG. Specific complexes at
x 400,000, bottom two rows sketched below.

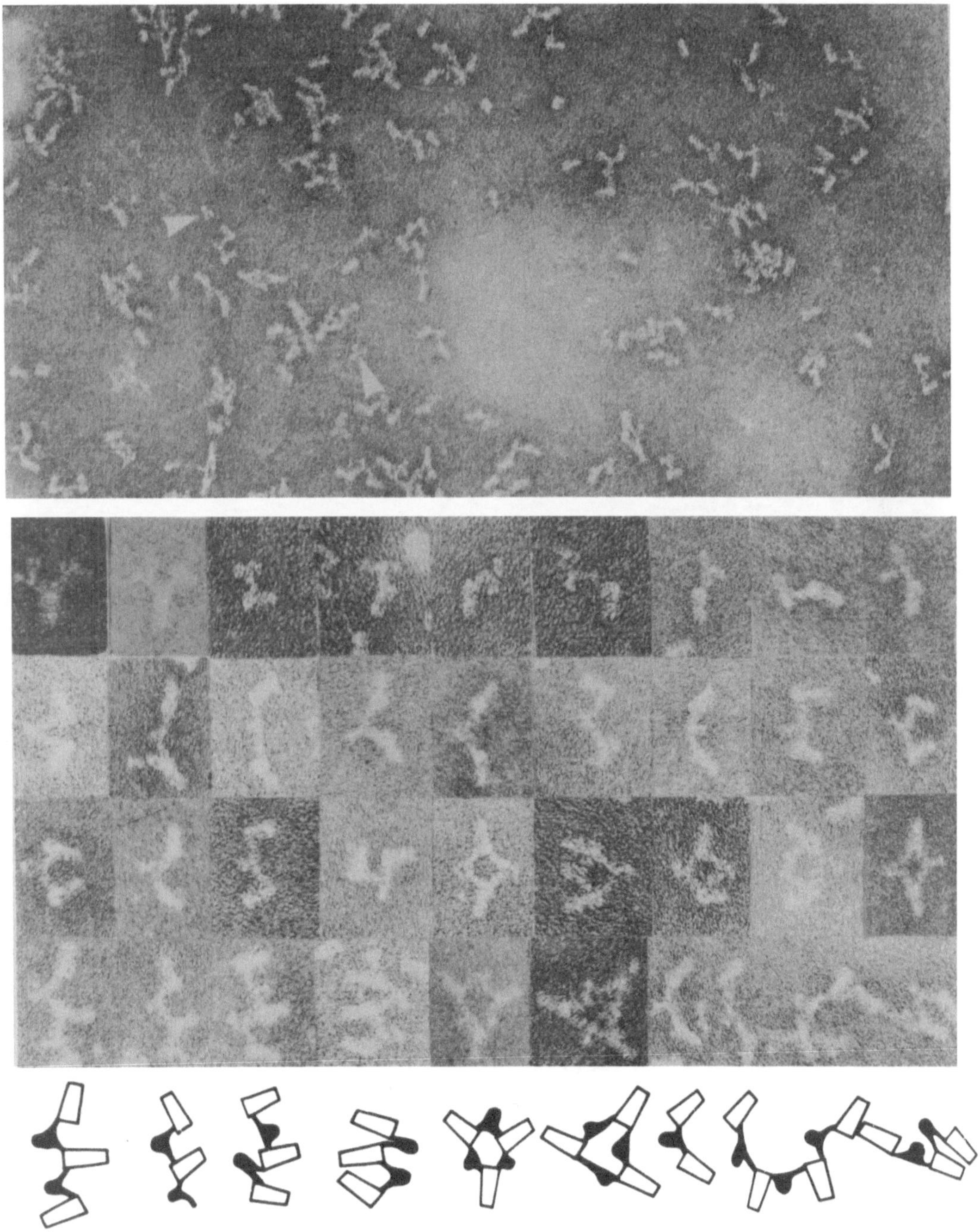

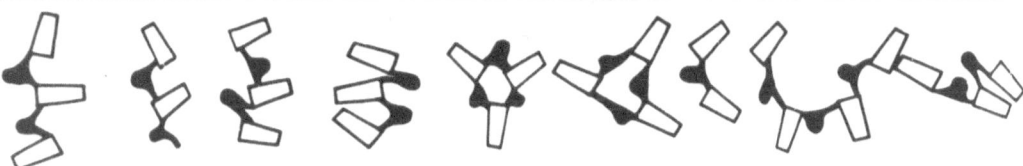

Figure 3

Incomplete hemagglutinin complexed with common antibody.

Top: General field at x 200,000, two free IgG molecules arrowed.

Center: Selected complexes at x 400,000. Note closed loops in third and fourth rows latter sketched below.

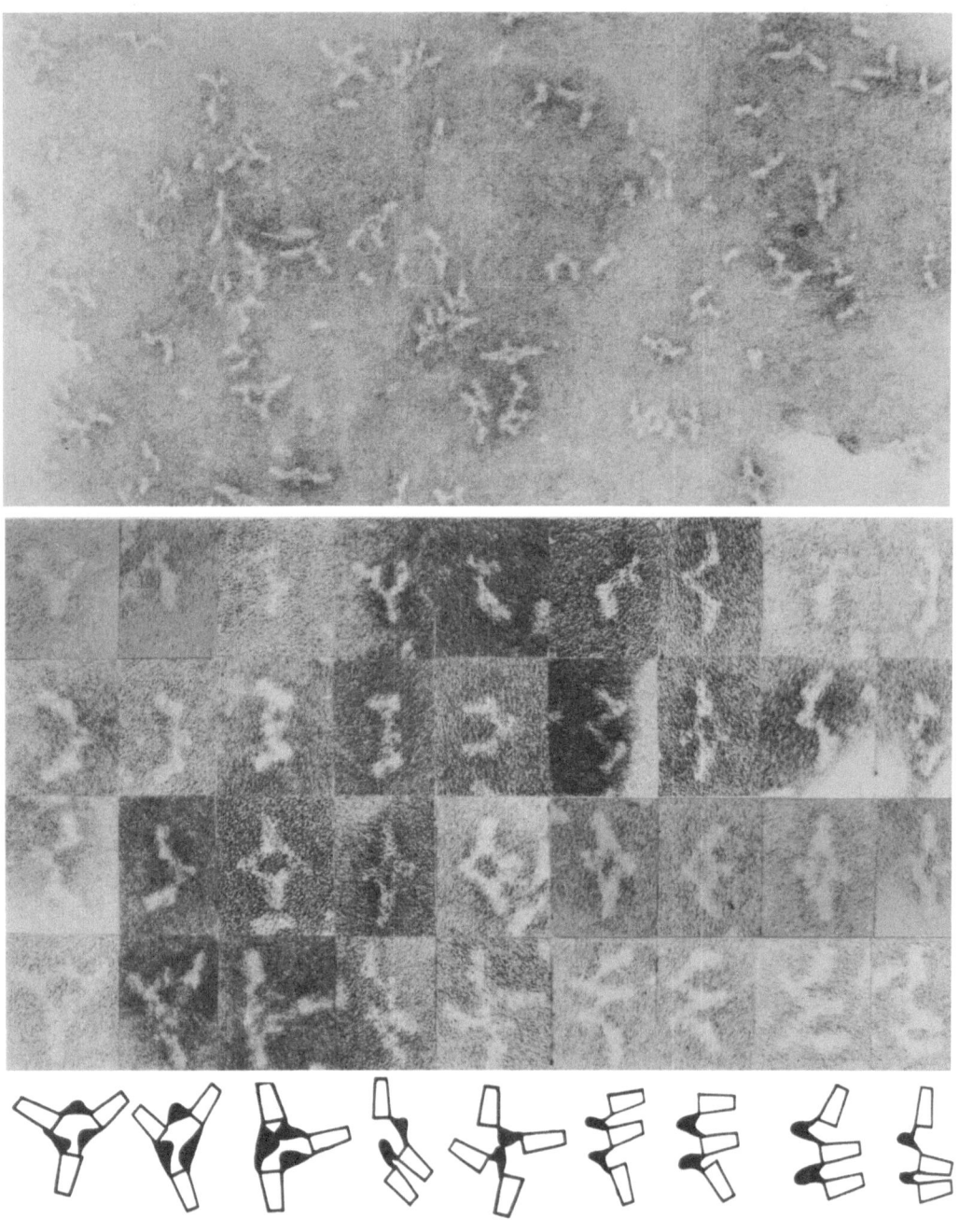

Figure 4

Incomplete hemagglutinin complexed with specific antibody.

Top: General field at x 200,000.

Center: Selected complexes at x 400,000, last row sketched below.

With complete hemagglutinin, the site of antibody binding was clearly and invariably near the distal end, apparently just down from the tip. Although there are probably other determinants along the length of the molecule, these would have been 'unavailable' to stimulate antibody production since the rabbit inoculum contained only aggregated rosettes of complete hemagglutinin. For this same reason, complexes with the incomplete hemagglutinin showed binding at one end only, presumed also to be the distal end.

All four figures show the binding of up to two antibody molecules per antigen *and never more*. This was surprising in view of the recent clear results of Wiley *et al.* (1977) showing that the hemagglutinin molecule is *trimeric*; each of its three identical subunits *must* carry the same antigenic determinants and should therefore bind up to three antibodies of any one type. There could be four reasons we did not observe the binding of three antibodies:

a. That complexes involving these bound antibodies would have been too tangled to interpret in the electron microscope; there were indeed some very large tangled complexes. However, in similar experiments with influenza neuraminidase (Wrigley *et al.*, 1977) which is tetrameric, we had no difficulty in observing three bound antibodies, and one instance of four.

b. That our empirical determination of the 'correct' proportions for mixing antigen and antibody (see Methods) was in fact outside the range in which three antibodies would bind. This seems statistically improbable, as we covered a very wide range of proportions.

c. That influenza hemagglutinin is in fact *dimeric*, possessing only two determinants of any one kind. This appears to be ruled out by the convincing results of Wiley *et al.* (1977).

d. That the third determinant is allosterically modified by binding antibody to the other two. Simple steric hinderance of third-site binding can be ruled out since the strict three-fold symmetry requirement for a trimer of three identical subunits would also prevent second-site binding. Thus allosteric modification of the third determinant seems the most likely reason we saw the binding of only two antibodies.

We did not attempt complexing of the hemagglutinin with both common and specific antibodies simultaneously. We have shown that the common and specific determinants are both close together (and may even overlap) at the distal end of the hemagglutin molecule so that binding of antibody to either would probably exclude the other. We have not determined relative affinities of the two types of binding, nor of the three determinants of each kind.

REFERENCES

BRAND, C. M. and SKEHEL, J. J. (1972) Nature New Biol. *238*, 145-147.

LAVER, W. G. (1969) In 'Fundamental Techniques in Virology' (Habel, K.and Saltzman, N. eds.), pp. 371-378, Academic Press, New York.

LAVER, W. G. and VALENTINE, R. C. (1969) Virology *38*, 105-119.

LAVER, W. G. and WEBSTER, R. G. (1973) Virology *51*, 383-391.

LAVER, W. G., DOWNIE, J. C. and WEBSTER, R. G. (1974) Virology *59*, 230-244.

SCHULZE, I. T. (1973) Advan. Virus Res. *18*, 1-55.

WILEY, D. C., SKEHEL, J. J. and WATERFIELD, M. D. (1977) Virology, in press.

WRIGLEY, N. G., LAVER, W. G. and DOWNIE, J. C. (1977) J. Mol. Biol. *109*, 405-421.

STUDIES ON THE STRUCTURE OF THE HEMAGGLUTININ

Don C. Wiley, Michael T. Flanagan, and John J. Skehel

There are two procedures in common use for the isolation of the hemagglutinin — one involves dissolution of virus particles with detergents, the other their digestion with proteases. As discussed elsewhere in this volume the former procedure yields the intact membrane glycoprotein (HA) which aggregates in the absence of detergent and, therefore, retains the ability to agglutinate erythrocytes. On the other hand, proteolytic digestion and more specifically bromelain digestion of virus particles (Brand and Skehel, 1972) results in the release of a soluble glycoprotein (BHA) which does not aggregate in detergent-free solution and is composed of hemagglutinin subunits which are modified at their carboxyl termini (Skehel and Waterfield, 1975). This report contains results of initial analyses of the three dimensional structure of the hemagglutinins prepared by these two different procedures and concerns X-ray diffraction studies of crystalline BHA and circular dichroism spectroscopy of HA and BHA.

a)   X-ray Diffraction

Several crystal forms have been observed during attempts to prepare crystals suitable for X-ray diffraction studies. BHA prepared from A/Weiss/43 (HO) formed octagonal plates in 1% polyethylene glycol 6000 and MRC-11 (H3) BHA formed hexagonal plates in 65% ammonium sulphate. These preparations have to date been too small for further analysis. X-31 (H3) BHA initially reported to form plates in water gives similar structures in 10% polyethylene glycol 6000. In addition larger (200μ) polycrystalline pentagonal dodecahedra were obtained from 65% ammonium sulphate pH 7.0 and octahedra up to 500μ edge dimension were grown from 80% sodium citrate pH 7.0 (Figure 1). The latter crystals are stable for at least 48 hours in the X-ray beam and are well ordered, diffracting out to 3 Å. They showed reciprocal lattice symmetry C4 with a systematic absence along c such that only spots for l=4n were present and this establishes the space group as tetragonal, $P4_1$ or $P4_3$. The unit cell dimensions are a=164Å, c=178Å. Crystal density measurements (Wiley and Skehel, 1977) indicate that two BHA molecules are present in each asymmetric unit of the crystal, X-ray data is being collected and heavy atom derivatives prepared.

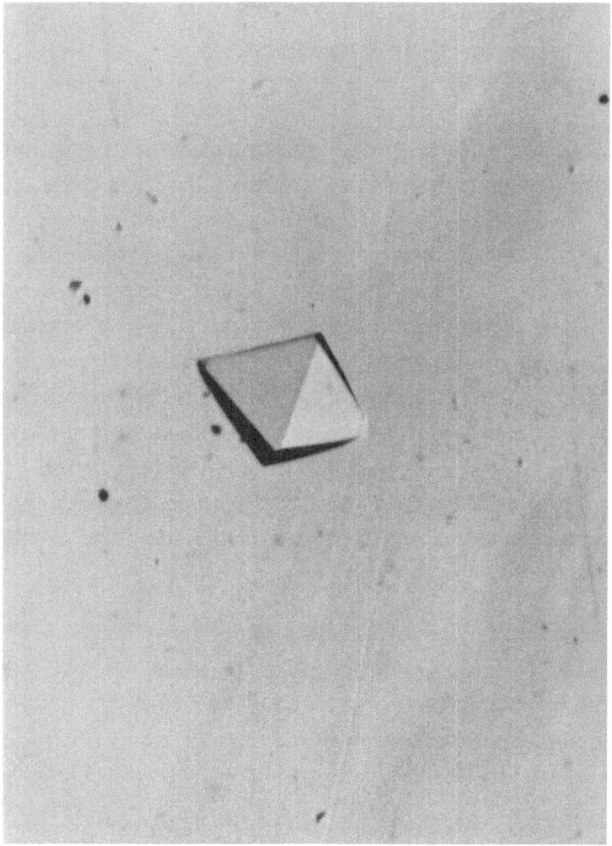

Figure 1
An octahedron of X-31 BHA formed in 80% sodium citrate, pH 7.0.

b)   Circular Dichroism

Since regular arrays of HA have not been observed diffraction studies are at present restricted to BHA preparations. The overall conformation of both molecular species in solution can, however, be compared by circular dichroism

spectroscopy and such analyses have been made in both the near and far ultraviolet between 300 and 190 nm. For these experiments BHA was prepared from
a variety of influenza viruses and in all cases similar results were obtained. Those
presented are for the hemagglutinin of A/Japan/305/57 (H2). HA was prepared
from virus particles of this strain by disrupting them in a 1.0% solution of the
non-ionic detergent Brij 36T. The results are shown in Figure 2 and Table 1.
Although the estimates of α-helix, β-structure and aperiodic structure obtained
from these experiments may be misleading as accurate predictions of structure
they are useful for comparative purposes. No difference within the experimental
error exists between the two spectra. The small differences observed, if significant, may reflect structure in the 'tail' peptide which was removed during
bromelain digestion (Brand and Skehel, 1972). Similarly the results of analyses
in the near UV (Figure 2) which reflect the asymmetric distribution within the
molecules of the amino acids tryptophan, tyrosine, phenylalanine and cysteine
also indicate that HA and BHA yield similar spectra. These similarities in both
the near and far UV CD spectra of HA and BHA therefore strongly suggest that
no major structural changes occur during bromelain digestion. More importantly
they imply that conclusions drawn from the results of studies on BHA will be
applicable to the intact membrane glycoprotein.

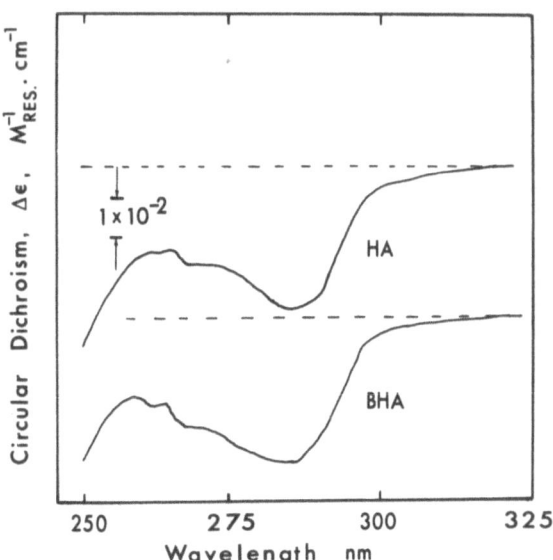

Figure 2
Near UV CD spectra of influenza virus hemagglutinin (A2/Japan/305/57).

Table 1

Analysis of the CD spectra (190-250 nm) of influenza virus hemagglutinin (A2/Japan/305/57) in terms of three contributing peptide conformations using the reference data of Chen, Yang and Martinez (1972)

Preparation	% Helix		% Beta Form		% Aperiodic Form	
HA	32.4	$\pm$1.2	14.0	$\pm$3.5	53.6	$\pm$9.5
BHA	29.4	$\pm$1.2	18.0	$\pm$3.9	52.6	$\pm$8.7

REFERENCES

BRAND, C. M. and SKEHEL, J. J. (1972) Nature N.B., *238*, 145-147.
SKEHEL, J. J. and WATERFIELD, M. D. (1975) Proc. Nat. Acad. Sci. U.S., *72*, 93-97.
WILEY, D. C. and SKEHEL, J. J. (1977) J. Mol. Biol. (In press).

PRELIMINARY STUDIES OF THE MEMBRANE-ASSOCIATED PORTION OF THE HEMAGGLUTININ

D. C. Wiley and J. J. Skehel

Like other 'intrinsic' membrane proteins the hemagglutinin is amphipathic. The results of comparative analyses of intact hemagglutinin molecules and preparations which lack the membrane associated hydrophobic region indicate that the portion of the molecule associated with the lipid bilayer is near the COOH-terminus of the smaller polypeptide component, HA_2 (Skehel and Waterfield, 1975).

In this communication two approaches to the detection and isolation of the membrane associated fragment are reported which are based on the hydrophobic characteristics expected of this portion of the molecule.

The isolation procedure is an application of the observations of Helenius and Simons (1977) that the electrophoretic mobilities of membrane proteins which bind detergent micelles are influenced by the charge of the micelle and may be manipulated by varying the type of detergent. In these experiments the cationic detergent cetyltrimethylammonium bromide and the nonionic detergent polyoxethylene 10-lauryl ether, Brij 36T were used. There were two sources of hemagglutinin protein — purified virus particles and plasma membranes from virus-infected chick embryo fibroblasts. Similar results were obtained using either source and the latter, in which the hemagglutinin polypeptide component was uncleaved biosynthetic precursor HA_0, was used in most experiments since the protein could be conveniently labelled in tissue culture using ^{35}S-methionine. The purification procedure used in the isolation of the radioactive hemagglutinin molecules from infected cell plasma membranes will be described in detail elsewhere but briefly it involved dissolution of the membranes in Brij 36T followed by sucrose density gradient centrifugation in solutions containing detergent. When such preparations in 0.5% Brij 36T were made with

respect to CTAB and electrophorezed at pH 8.6 in 1% agarose gels containing
the detergents in the same proportions, they migrated slightly towards the
cathode (Figure 1).

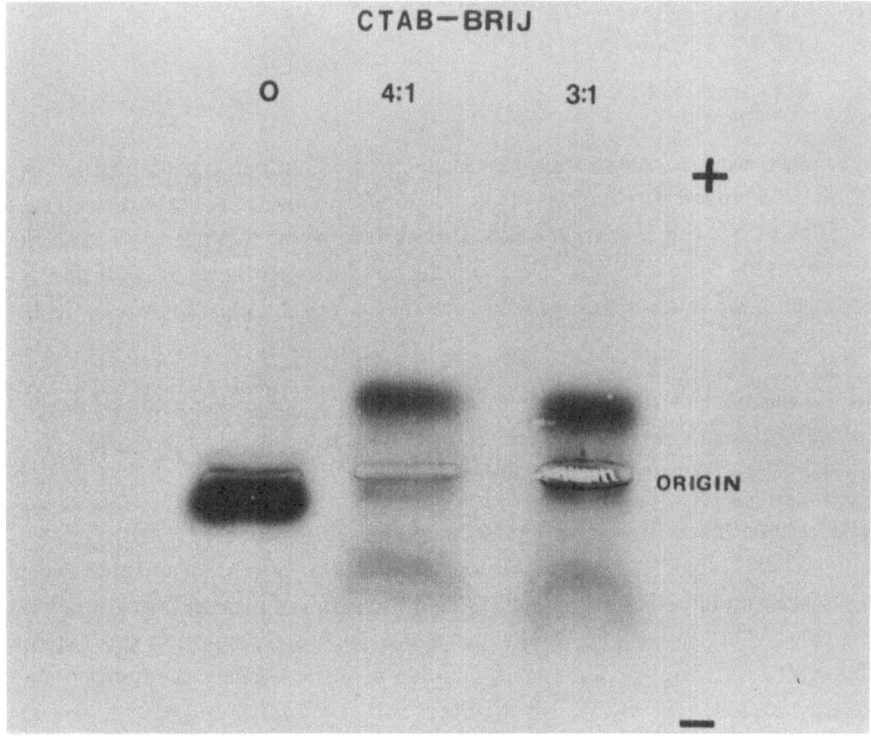

Figure 1

'Charge-shift' electrophoresis in agarose gels of the hemagglutinin before and after digestion
with bromelain. Lane 0 undigested HA_0 migrates as a cation. Lanes 4:1 and 3:1 (referring to
HA:bromelain ratio).
Bromelain digests of HA_0 at 37° for 3 hr. Electrophoresis was at 60 volts for 40 min. The
anionic material has been identified as BHA on agarose and by SDS-polyacrylamide gel
electrophoresis of bands cut from agarose gels. The light band near the origin is undigested
HA.
The cationic band which presumably binds the positively charged detergent micelles contains
peptides of molecular weight 5000-7000 as judged by the results of analyses on SDS-
polyacrylamide gels.

Bromelain digests of HA_0 are resolved into three components:

1. Near the origin, undigested HA_0 migrates as a cation.

2. The dominant component is an anion identified, by SDS polyacrylamide gel electrophoresis, as BHA – soluble bromelain released HA.

3. A cationic and probably, therefore, a detergent micelle-binding component. SDS-polyacrylamide gel electrophoretic analyses of this component indicate that its molecular weight is between 5000 and 7000. A similar low molecular weight component is found in CTAB-Brij/Agarose electrophoresis of bromelain-digested virus particles which have been pelleted and washed following digestion to remove soluble digestion products. These peptides which are probably derived from the hydrophobic region of the hemagglutinin molecule are the objects of further analyses.

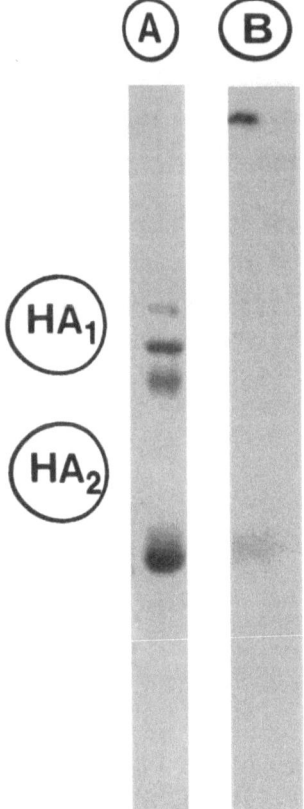

Figure 2

SDS-Polyacrylamide gel analysis of ^{125}I-nitrene labelled influenza virus. A. Virus polypeptides stained with Coomassie blue. B. Autoradiogram of A.

As stated above, for convenience the glycoprotein used in these studies was HA_0 labelled *in vivo* using ^{35}S-methionine. An alternative procedure which may be generally useful for labelling the lipid-associated regions of membrane proteins has also been investigated. Aryl azides have been utilized as photo-activateable reagents in several biological systems. In the present studies a diiodohexanoyl-derivative of 2-nitro, 4-azido phenyl tyramine prepared by M. Hebden and J. Knott, which partitioned preferentially before activation into the lipid bilayer of virus particles was used to label the lipid and lipid-associated virus protein molecules. The results of the procedure can be assessed following separation of the SDS-dissociated virus polypeptides by polyacrylamide gel electrophoresis (Figure 2). The smaller polypeptide of the hemagglutinin, HA_2, was clearly the most highly labelled virus component and since, as mentioned above, the COOH-terminal portion of HA_2 has been implicated as the lipid associated part of the molecule it appears likely that this region is specifically labelled.

An important practical implication of this result is of course that the hemagglutinin of large quantities of egg-grown virus can be labelled *in vitro* and preparation of the hydrophobic 'tails' from the labelled molecules should facilitate their detailed analysis.

REFERENCES

SKEHEL, J. J. and WATERFIELD, M. D. (1975). Proc. Nat. Acad. Sci. U.S., *72*, 93-97.
HELENIUS, A. and SIMONS, K. (1977) Proc. Nat. Acad. Sci. USA. *74*, 529-532.

’N-TERMINAL AMINO ACID ANALYSIS OF HEMAGGLUTININ
MOLECULES FROM DUCK AND EQUINE INFLUENZA VIRUSES
PREVIOUSLY IMPLICATED AS PROGENITORS OF THE HONG KONG
STRAIN OF HUMAN INFLUENZA

W. G. Laver and R. G. Webster

Summary

The hemagglutinin molecules from a number of strains of influenza virus, including those of
the Asian (H2N2) series, have been found to possess N-terminal aspartic acid (or asparagine)
at the N-terminus of the large polypeptide (HA_1). The only virus strains found so far which
do not possess N-terminal aspartic acid on the hemagglutinin are those of the Hong Kong
(H3N2) series, where the N-terminus seems to be blocked.

We have found that the hemagglutinin molecules of equine-2 (Heq2Neq2) and duck/Ukraine
(Hav7Neq2) viruses also lack N-terminal aspartic acid. This finding is consistant with the idea
that the hemagglutinin molecules of Hong Kong influenza virus were derived, by genetic recombination, from a virus related to equine-2 and duck/Ukraine viruses and that they did not
arise by mutation of an Asian (H2N2) influenza virus.

Influenza viruses infecting man undergo, at periodic intervals, major antigenic
shifts. In these shifts, sudden and complete changes occur in one or both of the
surface antigens so that 'new' viruses arise to which the population has no immunity, and it is these viruses which cause pandemic influenza.

The way in which these 'new' viruses arise is not known, but evidence has been
obtained which suggests that one 'new' virus, Hong Kong 1968 strain (H3N2),
may have been formed as the result of genetic recombination between an
'Asian' (H2N2) virus and an animal or bird influenza virus related to equine-2
and duck/Ukraine viruses (for a review, see Webster and Laver, 1975).

The neuraminidase molecules of Hong Kong influenza and Asian influenza were
found to be similar, but the hemagglutinin molecules of these two viruses were
unrelated antigenically, and tryptic peptide maps of the two polypeptides of
the hemagglutinin showed many differences between the two strains. These

findings suggested that the hemagglutinin of Hong Kong influenza did not arise by mutation of an Asian Virus.

The hemagglutinin molecules of Hong Kong influenza were found to be antigenically related to those of equine-2 and duck/Ukraine viruses which were isolated in 1963, five years before Hong Kong influenza appeared in man. Furthermore, maps of tryptic peptides of one of the hemagglutinin polypeptides (HA_2) from Hong Kong influenza were similar to maps of HA_2 from equine-2 and duck/Ukraine viruses, suggesting that all three viruses had a common progenitor.

We have now found a further structural similarity between the hemagglutinin molecules of Hong Kong influenza and those of equine-2 and duck/Ukraine viruses.

The hemagglutinin molecules of influenza virus are formed from a single kind of precursor polypeptide (HA) which is cleaved during virus maturation into two polypeptides — a large one (HA_1) and a small one (HA_2).

The N-terminal amino acid of the large polypeptide (HA_1) is aspartic acid (or asparagine) in the case of the following viruses: X-38 (Heq1), BEL (H0), Weiss (H1), Singapore/57 (H2) and Turkey/Mass (Hav6). In addition, the hemagglutinin molecules (containing both HA_1 and HA_2) of the following viruses have been shown to possess N-terminal aspartic acid, and in these cases it is also probably on HA_1: PR8 (H0), MEL (H0), FM1 (H1), Nederlands/68 (H2), Shearwater virus (Hav6) and B/LEE (Laver, 1962, 1964; Skehel and Waterfield, 1975; Bucher *et al.*, 1976). The only strain of influenza virus found so far which does not possess N-terminal aspartic acid on the hemagglutinin is Hong Kong influenza (H3N2) and its antigenic variants. The amino acid at the N-terminus of Hong Kong HA_1 has not been identified and may be blocked (Ward, personal communication). The N-terminus of HA_2 which is formed as the result of cleavage of the HA precursor polypeptide is glycine, in all influenza virus strains so far examined.

The question we asked therefore was: 'Do the viruses which we think donated the hemagglutinin during the formation of Hong Kong influenza (equine/2 and duck/Ukraine) possess N-terminal aspartic acid on HA_1, or is the N-terminus blocked? '

Hemagglutinin molecules from the following strains of type A influenza were therefore analysed for N-terminal amino acids: A/Nederlands/84/68 (H2N2), A/Port Chalmers/73 (H3N2), A/Victoria/75 (H3N2), A/Shearwater/E. Aust./72 (Hav6Nav5), A/equine/Miami/1/63 (Heq2Neq2), A/duck/Ukraine/1/63 (Hav7 Neq2) and A/BEL/42 (H0N1).

Recombinant influenza viruses (antigenic hybrids) possessing the neuraminidase molecules of the A/BEL/42 (H0N1) strain of influenza virus and the hemagglutinin molecules of the above viruses were prepared as previously described (Webster, 1970). The recombinant viruses were grown in the allantoic sac of 11-day-old chick embryos and the virus particles were purified by adsorption-elution on erythrocytes followed by differential centrifugation and sedimentation through a sucrose gradient (10-40% sucrose in 0.15 M NaCl) as previously described (Laver, 1969).

Isolation of the Hemagglutinin Molecules

The virus particles were disrupted with 1% sodium dodecyl sulfate (SDS) at room temperature (20°C) and the virus proteins were separated by electrophoresis on cellulose acetate strips in Tris-boric acid-EDTA buffer pH 9 containing 0.4% SDS as previously described (Laver and Webster, 1973).

Separation of the Light and Heavy Chains of the Hemagglutinin

The hemagglutinin molecules, isolated as described above, were precipitated with cold (-20°C) ethanol (66% v/v), drained until free of excess ethanol and redissolved by heating to 100°C in saturated guanidine hydrochloride solution (0.3 ml) containing dithiothreitol (0.5 mg/ml). The light and heavy polypeptide chains were then separated by centrifuging on guanidine hydrochloride-dithiothreitol density gradients as previously described (Laver and Webster, 1973).

N-Terminal Amino Acid Analysis

The isolated hemagglutinin molecules or the large polypeptide of the hemagglutinin (HA_1) were precipitated with 60% ethanol, redissolved in saturated guanidine hydrochloride solution and heated to 100° for 1 minute. After cooling, $NaHCO_3$ (1%) was added and excess 2,4-dinitro-1-fluorobenzene. The mix-

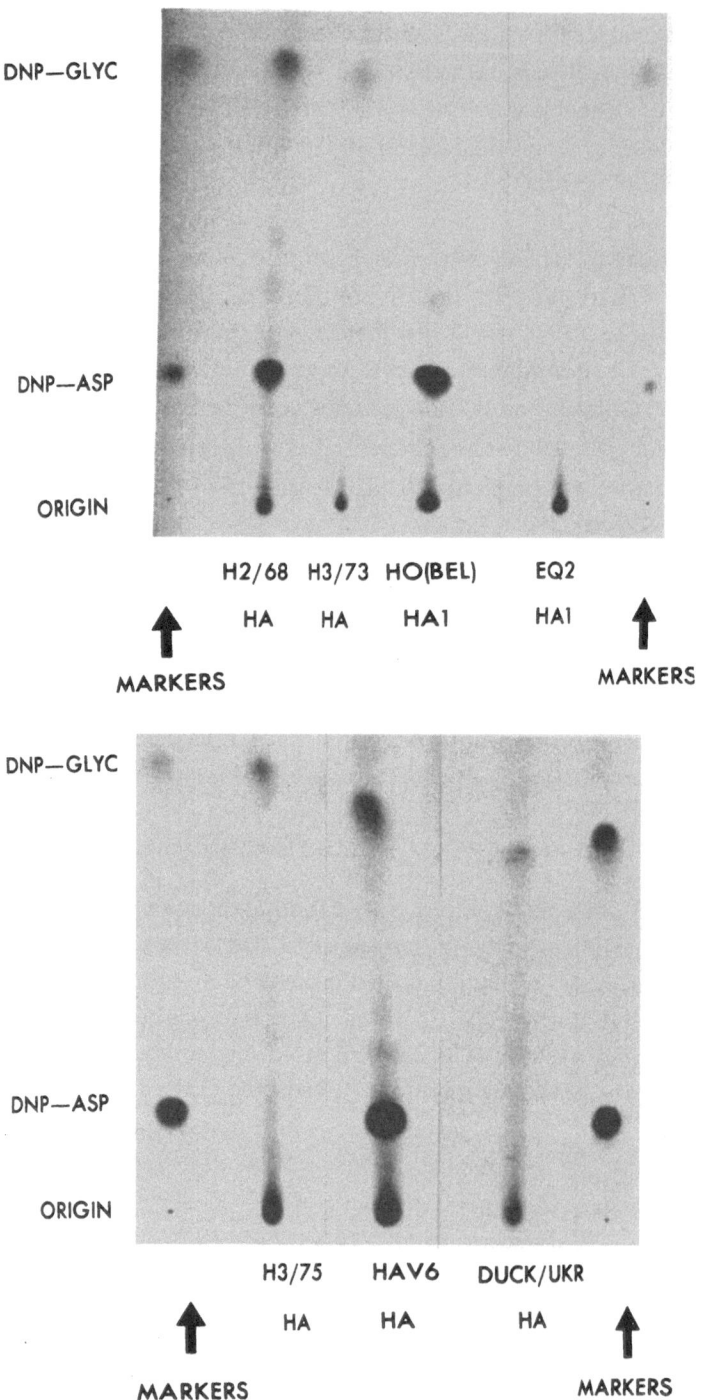

ture was incubated with occasional shaking for 6 hours at $37^{\circ}C$. The DNP-proteins were then precipitated with ethanol, washed with ethanol and a mixture of chloroform-methanol (2:1) and dried. The DNP-proteins were then hydrolysed in 6N HCl in sealed, evacuated tubes for 22 hours at 110°. The hydrolysed DNP-proteins were diluted to bring the HCl concentration to about 1N and extracted three times with ether. The ether extracts were pooled, taken to dryness and the DNP-amino acids were dissolved in methanol and separated by polyamide thin-layer chromatography according to Wang *et al.*, 1966. The chromatograms were photographed using a blue filter. The aqueous phase was not examined.

The results obtained are shown in Figure 1. DNP-aspartic acid was obtained from the hemagglutinin molecules of Nederlands/68 (H2N2) and Shearwater/72 (Hav6Nav5) viruses and from HA_1 of A/BEL/42 (H0N1) virus.

Neither of the Hong Kong strains, A/Port Chalmers/73 (H3N2) or A/Victoria/75 (H3N2) possessed N-terminal aspartic acid on the hemagglutinin, though DNP-glycine derived from the N-terminus of HA_2 was present.

It can be clearly seen from Figure 1 that neither equine-2 HA_1 nor duck/Ukraine HA possessed free N-terminal aspartic acid, though in the latter case N-terminal glycine was present, presumably on HA_2. Equine-2 HA molecules also possessed N-terminal glycine (not shown in Figure 1).

These findings are consistant with the suggestion which we made from the result of peptide mapping experiments (Laver and Webster, 1973), that the

---

Figure 1

Photographs of thin-layer chromatograms of the ether-soluble DNP-amino acids obtained by hydrolysis of the DNP-substituted hemagglutinin molecule (containing HA_1 and HA_2) or the hemagglutinin large polypeptide (HA_1) from a number of strains of influenza virus.

H2/68 = A/Nederlands/84/68 (H2N2), H3/73 = A/Port Chalmers/73 (H3N2), H0 (BEL) = A/BEL/42 (H0N1), Eq2 = A/equine/Miami/1/63 (Heq2Neq2), H3/75 = A/Victoria/75 (H3N2), Hav6 = A/Shearwater/E. Aust./72 (Hav6Nav5) and DUCK/UKR = A/duck/Ukraine/1/63 (Hav7Neq2).

The DNP-amino acids were chromatographed on polyamide thin-layer plates (Wang *et al.*, 1966) in benzene-glacial acetic acid, 80:20 v/v. Three rounds of ascending chromatography with drying in between were used. The yellow spots were photographed through a blue filter.

'new' hemagglutinin subunits of the virus which arose in 1968 (A/Hong Kong/ 68, H3N2) came by genetic recombination from an animal or bird influenza virus related to equine-2 and duck/Ukraine viruses, and that they did not arise by mutation of an Asian (H2N2) influenza virus strain.

Acknowledgements

Jean Clark and Donna Cameron provided excellent technical assistance. This work was supported in part by research grant AI08831 from the National Institute of Allergy and Infectious Diseases to R.G.W. The suggestion to look for N-terminal aspartic acid on equine-2 and duck/Ukraine hemagglutinin molecules was made by Dr. Colin Ward.

REFERENCES

BUCHER, D. J., LI, S. S-L., KEHOE, J. M. and KILBOURNE, E. D. (1976) Proc. Nat. Acad. Sci. USA. *73*, 238-242.

LAVER, W. G. (1962) Virology *18*, 19-32.

LAVER, W. G. (1964) J. Mol. Biol. *9*, 109-124.

LAVER, W. G. (1969) in 'Fundamental Techniques in Virology' (Habel, K. and Salzman, N. eds.) pp. 82, Academic Press, New York.

LAVER, W. G. and WEBSTER, R. G. (1973) Virology *51*, 383-391.

SKEHEL, J. J. and WATERFIELD, M. D. (1975) Proc. Nat. Acad. Sci. USA. *72*, 93-97.

WANG, K. T., HUANG, J. M. K. and WANG, I. S. Y. (1966) J. Chromatog. *22*, 362-368.

WEBSTER, R. G. (1970) Virology *42*, 633-642.

WEBSTER, R. G. and LAVER, W. G. (1975) in 'The Influenza Viruses and Influenza' (Kilbourne, E. D., ed.) pp. 269, Academic Press, New York.

THE CHEMISTRY OF ANTIGENIC VARIATION IN INFLUENZA A VIRUS HEMAGGLUTININ

B. A. Moss and P. Anne Underwood

Summary

Single-step antigenic mutants, derived experimentally from the strain A/NT60/68 (H3N2), have been used to study the chemistry of antigenic variation within the present subtype of influenza A virus. These mutants mimic the antigenic drift of field strains that arose naturally between 1968 and 1973. Hemagglutinin, the major viral coat antigen, was prepared free of neuraminidase by controlled digestion of each virus strain with the protease, bromelain. The antigenic reactivity of the hemagglutinin was not altered by this treatment.

The hemagglutinin preparations, after reduction and S-alkylation, were digested with trypsin and compared by fluorescent dansyl-peptide mapping on thin layers of silica gel. This sensitive mapping technique, operating on a nanomole of protein, permitted resolution of virtually all the tryptic peptides.

The maps of all strains were identical, except for one or two peptides migrating differently. The variable peptides were confined to the larger subunit (HA_1) of the hemagglutinin molecule. Thus, variation within a hierarchic series of antigenic mutants is associated with minor changes in the primary structure of the larger hemagglutinin subunit. Since the strains examined differed only in their antigenic properties, it is likely that the variable peptide in which amino acid substitutions occurred formed part of the antigenic determinant.

Introduction

The viruses of influenza are variable, as has been demonstrated soon after isolation of the first human strain (Francis and Shope, 1936; Magill and Francis, 1936; Smorodintseff et al., 1936) and repeatedly confirmed thereafter. The most extensive and epidemiologically most relevant variation concerns the hemagglutinin molecule, one of the glycoproteins making up the viral coat.

Even though the hemagglutinin molecule has been subject to extensive protein-chemical studies (Laver and Webster, 1968,1971,1973; Webster and Laver, 1971; Laver et al., 1974; Laver, 1973) the site of antigenic variation could not be defined, partly because many of the tryptic peptides remained as an insoluble core and partly because each of the field strains tested differed in several peptides.

The aim of this study was to establish a technique which allows complete resolution of tryptic peptides from the hemagglutinin molecule, and then apply it to a set of isogenic mutants, differing only in their antigenic properties (Fazekas de St. Groth, 1969a,b,1970,1975,1977; Fazekas de St. Groth and Hannoun, 1973).

Experimental Procedures

Virus Strains

The antigenic mutants were selected under the pressure of antibody from the strain A/NT60/68 (H3N2) by Fazekas de St. Groth (1969a,b,1970,1975,1977; Fazekas de St. Groth and Hannoun, 1973). The parental strain A/NT60/68 and its single-step antigenic mutants 375/17, 29C, 142/6 and 30C, which were examined in this study, were provided by Dr. Fazekas de St. Groth. Their genetic relationship is described in this volume.

Indicator Virus

Indicator virus was prepared from influenza strain A/PR8/34 (H0N0) using the method of Stone (1949).

Purification of Virus

All viruses were propagated in the allantois of 11 day old chick embryos. They were partially purified and concentrated by adsorption-elution on fowl erythrocytes, followed by high-speed centrifugation, to give a preparation containing 50 mg virus/ml.

Further purification was carried out by two stages of sucrose density gradient centrifugation (Reimer *et al.*, 1966) in a Beckman Ti-15 zonal rotor. The kinetic run (1350ml sucrose, 20-35%, equivolumetric gradient) was done at 20,000 rpm for 1 hr. The isopycnic gradient (1200ml sucrose, 35-50%, linear) was spun for 20-22 hr at 30,000 rpm. Fractions containing the peak of purified virus (see Figure 1) were pooled, spun down, and resuspended in HAS to a concentration of 5×10^5 HAU per ml (8.33 mg virus protein/ml).

Monitoring Methods for Hemagglutinin Production

Hemagglutinating Activity

Hemagglutinating activity was measured by the method of Fazekas de St. Groth (1955). A hemagglutinating unit (HAU) is that amount of virus which gives the conventional endpoint against 1 ml of 1% fowl erythrocytes, bridging 15.3% of the cells (Fazekas de St. Groth and Cairns, 1952).

Antibody-blocking Test

The test (Fazekas de St. Groth to be published) was carried out in Microtiter trays in 0.1 ml volumes. Serial two-fold dilutions of the test preparations were made in 0.025 ml HAS. An equal volume of homologous hyperimmune rabbit serum, containing 3 inhibitory units of antibody, was added to each and the mixture left at room temperature for 1 hr. Then 0.025 ml 1% fowl erythrocytes were added, followed immediately by o.025 ml HAS containing 3 agglutinating units of homologous whole virus and the test read after 30 min incubation at room temperature. This test can detect 0.01 μg of hemagglutinin.

Neuraminidase Activity

Neuraminidase activity was measured as described by Stone (1949). Serial two-fold dilutions of the test sample were made in 0.25 ml CaMg saline in glass tubes and 0.025 ml of ovomucin solution, containing 4 inhibitory units, was added to each tube. After incubation for 1 hr at 35°C the tubes were heated at 62.5°C for 10 min to destroy hemagglutinin and any further enzyme activity. The tubes were cooled to room temperature and inhibitory activity of residual ovomucin was titrated by the method of Fazekas de St. Groth (1952).

The above titrations were all performed in duplicate.

Polyacrylamide Gel Electrophoresis

Polyacrylamide gel electrophoresis in sodium dodecyl sulphate (SDS) was based on the method of Laemmli (1970) as modified by Underwood (to be published) and performed in Gradipore equipment (Margolis and Kenrick, 1968). The gel slab (10% acrylamide + 0.3% BIS) contained no SDS and was made up in 0.3 M Tris-glycine, pH 8.5 to give improved staining with Coomassie Brilliant Blue R250 (CBB). The electrode buffer (pH 8.5) contained 0.05 M glycine; 0.007 M Tris; 0.1% SDS and 0.08% sodium azide and was maintained at 7-9°C during runs. Samples containing 2% SDS, 5% 2-mercaptoethanol, 10% glycerol, 0.002% bromocresol purple and 0.1 M Tris phosphate buffer pH 6.8, were heated in boiling water for 2 min immediately prior to loading. Usually 2 to 20 μg of protein were analyzed.

Electrophoresis was carried out at 80 volts and 20 mamp per gel for 4 hr. Gels were stain/fixed in 0.5% CBB in 30% methanol, 10% sulphosalicylic acid, 5% trichloracetic acid for 2 hr at room temperature and destained overnight in 30% methanol, 7% acetic acid. Gels for carbohydrate staining were fixed and stained by the PAS method of Kapitany and Zebrowski (1973).

The gels were sliced vertically and scanned in a Gilford spectrophotometer fitted with a linear transport mechanism (570 nm wavelength for CBB and 560 for PAS). Using these methods 0.5 μg carbohydrate can be detected.

Preparation of Hemagglutinin from Purified Virus Particles

External proteins on the virus surface (neuraminidase and hemagglutinin) were removed in a two stage process involving the protease, bromelain (Fazekas de St. Groth and Forster, 1973). Bromelain concentrations were adjusted for each virus strain and averaged 0.06 mg/ml for Stage 1 and 0.02 mg/ml for Stage 2.

Stage 1

Equal volumes of bromelain preparation and virus suspension (8.33 mg/ml virus protein) were mixed at $4^{\circ}C$ and maintained at this temperature, with occasional shaking, for 2 hr. The mixture was then tested for hemagglutinating activity and centrifuged at 70,000 g for 30 min at $4^{\circ}C$. The pellet ('semi-cores') was resuspended in the original volume of HAS and used for Stage 2. The supernatant was applied to a column of Sephadex G100 superfine (1.6 cm x 24 cm), eluted at 20 ml/hr with 0.1 M ammonium bicarbonate buffer, pH 7.8. Column effluents were monitored at 280 nm through a Uvicord 1 spectrophotometer and collected in 3 ml fractions. The excluded peak contained neuraminidase.

Stage 2

An equal volume of bromelain preparation was added to the resuspended pellet, and the mixture incubated at $35^{\circ}C$ for 2 hr with occasional shaking. It was then tested for hemagglutinating activity, chilled to arrest enzyme action, and centrifuged at 75,000 g for 45 min at $4^{\circ}C$. The pellet ('cores') was resuspended in the original volume of HAS. The supernatant was filtered through Sephadex, as above. The excluded peak contained the antigenically intact hemagglutinin, which was stored frozen or freeze-dried under nitrogen at $-20^{\circ}C$ until required for peptide analysis.

Reduction and Alkylation of Hemagglutinin

Complete reduction and alkylation of hemagglutinin (HA) preparations was performed in denaturing buffer (7 M GuHCl-0.5 M Tris acetate-2 mM EDTA, pH 8.5) at protein concentrations ranging from 0.1 to 4 mg/100 μl. Usually 0.2 mg was used. The HA in 75 μl was reduced under nitrogen for 1 hr at $50^{\circ}C$ by addition of dithiothreitol dissolved in 25 μl of denaturing buffer (1.75-70 μmoles DTT or 100-fold molar excess over protein -SH). After reduction, the DTT concentration was quickly lowered by precipitating the protein with cold ($-20^{\circ}C$) absolute ethanol (1 ml) acidified with glacial acetic acid (10 μl). After 30 min at $-20^{\circ}C$ the flocculent protein was sedimented by centrifugation (1,500 x g/10 min) and washed with cold ($-20^{\circ}C$) 70% ethanol containing DTT (1 x 1 ml; 0.02-0.8 mM DTT dependent on protein concentration). The precipitate was redissolved in 75 μl of denaturing buffer containing DTT (17.5-700 nmoles to give equimolar amounts of DTT and protein -SH). The HA was then alkylated under nitrogen at $25^{\circ}C$ in the dark with iodo[2-^{14}C]acetic acid dissolved in

25 μl of denaturing buffer (iodoacetic acid 25 μ Ci/μmole; 0.1-4 μmole or about 3-fold molar excess over total -SH concentration). The alkylation was stopped after 1 hr by quenching with an excess of 2-mercaptoethanol (10 μl) followed by 10 μl of glacial acetic acid to lower the pH to about 5. The carboxymethyl-ated preparations (CM-HA) were either applied to a column which separates the two hemagglutinin subunits, or were desalted by precipitation with cold absolute ethanol as before and washed with cold 70% ethanol (3 x 1 ml).

In some cases the reduced hemagglutinin was alkylated with unlabelled iodo-acetic acid or iodoacetamide.

Separation of the Hemagglutinin Subunits

The reduced or reduced,S-carboxymethylated hemagglutinin (0.4 - 4 mg) was fractionated at 20°C by molecular exclusion chromatography on columns of Bio-gel P150 (Bio-Rad Laboratories, 100-200 mesh, 1.6 cm x 65 cm) equilibrat-ed with 6 M GuHCl - 0.05 M sodium acetate - 0.001 M DTT, pH 5.0 (Green and Bolognesi, 1974).

The flow rate was 2.4 ml/hr, and 1.2 ml fractions were collected. The appropri-ate protein-containing fractions were pooled, dialyzed thoroughly against sev-eral changes of 0.005 M ammonium hydroxide at 4°C, and then freeze-dried.

Amino Acid Analysis and NH$_2$-Terminal Sequences

CM-HA samples (50 - 100 μg) were hydrolyzed at 110°C in 0.2 ml of redistilled constant-boiling HCl, containing phenol (0.1 mg/ml) and 2-mercaptoethanol (0.1% v/v), in evacuated, sealed Pyrex glass tubes for 24, 48, and 72 hr. The hydrolysates were dried *in vacuo* over NaOH pellets to remove HCl. The dried samples were dissolved in 2 ml of 0.01 N HCl and 1 ml aliquots, analyzed with a dual column Jeolco JLC-6AH automatic amino acid analyzer equipped with high sensitivity 10 mm cuvettes and electronically expanded recorder range. L-Norleucine and α-amino-β-guanidinopropionic acid (each 5 nmole/ml) were included in sample dilutor to serve as internal standards.

Freeze-dried CM-HA preparations (2-4 nmoles) were dissolved in 0.2 ml of 0.5 M sodium bicarbonate coupling buffer, pH 9.8 and 20 μl of 10% (w/v) SDS solution. Amino terminal sequence analyses were performed according to the manual SDS-dansyl-Edman procedure of Weiner *et al.* (1972) except that the phenyl thiocarbamyl hemagglutinin derivatives were precipitated with acetone rendered 1 mM in 2-mercaptoethanol.

Tryptic Peptide Maps

For tryptic digestion CM-HA (200 μg) was suspended in distilled water (0.1 ml) and warmed for 2 min in a boiling water bath. Then 0.2 M triethylamine bicarbonate buffer, pH 8.5 (0.1ml) was added. Trypsin-TPCK (Worthington Biochemical Corp., 1 μg in 2 μl of 1 mM HCl-2.5 mM CaCl$_2$) was added and the mixture incubated under nitrogen at 37°C. (The flocculent suspension usually cleared within 1 hr). After 2 hr an additional 2 μl of trypsin-TPCK was added and incubation continued for another 4 hr.

The tryptic peptides were dansylated by a procedure (Moss, 1977) adapted from the methods of Zanetta *et al.* (1970) and Tamura *et al.* (1973). Briefly, dansylation was effected in 0.1 M triethylamine with an equal volume of 20 mM dansyl chloride in acetone (100 moles per mole peptide) for 2 hr at 37°C. The apparent pH of the mixture was about 10.5. Recovery of the dansyl-peptides was essentially according to the method of Zanetta *et al.* (1970). Fingerprinting of the dansyl-peptides (from 0.5 - 1 nmole HA preparation) was achieved by two-dimensional chromatography on Silica gel G (Merck, Type 60), spread as a 0.3 mm layer over glass plates (20 cm x 20 cm). Development was done at 20°C in the dark for 1.5 hr in the first dimension (methylacetate-isopropanol-25% ammonia; 9:6:4 by vol.), and 3.5 hr in the second dimension (isobutanol-acetic acid-water; 15:4:2 by vol.). The plates were quickly dried in a warm air stream, viewed under long wavelength ultraviolet light (Chromato-Vue Mineralight, Calif., USA.) and the fluorescent spots rapidly outlined to avoid excessive photochemical-degradation. Peptides were removed from the plates according to Gros (1967), and eluted from the small chromatotubes with acetone-water-acetic acid-pyridine (50:50:1:3 by vol.), (Tamura *et al.*, 1973)

Results

Isolation of Hemagglutinin

Highly purified virus particles were obtained using the successive rate zonal (kinetic) and isopycnic sucrose density gradient centrifugations described (Figure 1). These virus particles were used in the release of neuraminidase and hemagglutinin sequentially from the viral envelope with bromelain. Bromelain concentrations were adjusted for each virus strain to (a) maximize removal of neuraminidase and minimize removal of hemagglutinin in Stage 1 of the preparative procedures, and (b) maximize removal of antigenically active hemagglutinin in Stage 2. The average bromelain concentrations used were 0.06 mg/ml for Stage 1 and 0.02 mg/ml for Stage 2 which gave considerably lower enzyme: viral protein substrate ratios (1:140 and 1:400 respectively) than the ratio of 1:2 described by Brand and Skehel (1972).

Filtration of the supernatant from Stage 1 through Sephadex G100, revealed two U.V. absorbing fractions (Figure 2A). The excluded peak contained a

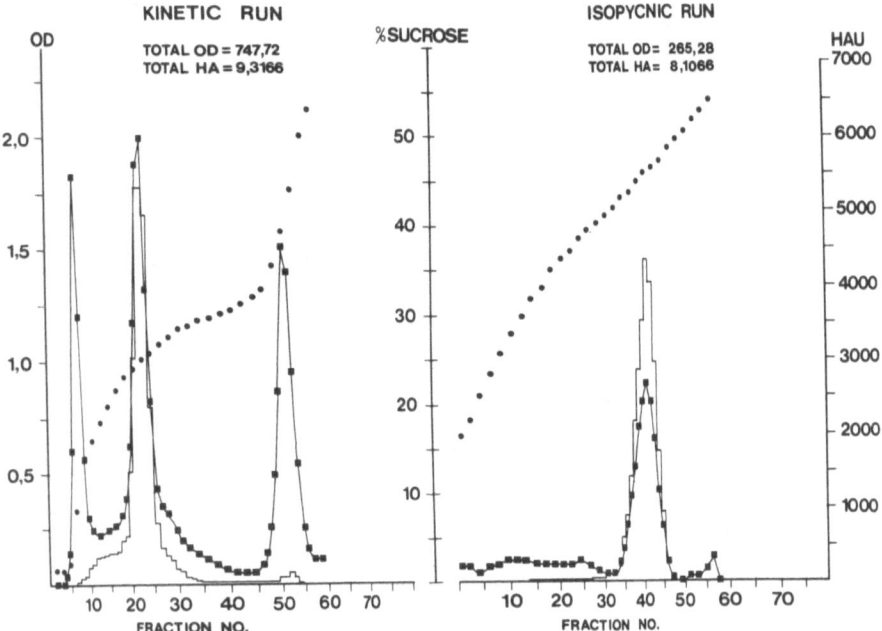

Figure 1

Sucrose Density Gradient Purification of Influenza Virus Strain A3/NT60

Virus particles were purified by two steps of sucrose density gradient centrifugation. The rate-zonal (kinetic) gradient was spun at 20,000 rpm for 1 hr in the Beckman titanium-15 zonal rotor. The isopycnic gradient was spun for 20-22 hr at 30,000 rpm. Uvicord I absorbance (O.D.), ■————■ ; sucrose concentration, ... ; the histogram represents hemagglutinating activity.

protein with the mobility of neuraminidase on SDS-polyacrylamide gels (Figure 3) and exhibiting a positive PAS-reaction, but no neuraminidase activity. Low levels of hemagglutinin antibody blocking activity were sometimes observed, together with faint PAS-positive bands corresponding in position to hemagglutinin on SDS-gels. The excluded peak was well separated from bromelain and breakdown products, eluted immediately before the buffer salts. Figure 2B illustrates the elution profile of the supernatant from Stage 2. The excluded peak contained a PAS-positive protein corresponding to hemagglutinin on SDS-gels (Figure 3). A high level of antibody blocking activity was evident (Figure 2B) but no hemagglutinin activity. No virus proteins other than hemagglutinin were ever detected. The smaller subunit (HA_2) of this hemagglutinin showed a higher mobility on SDS-gels than its counterpart in native whole virus (Figure 3), as has been demonstrated previously for bromelain-cleaved hemagglutinin

FILTRATION ON G100 SEPHADEX

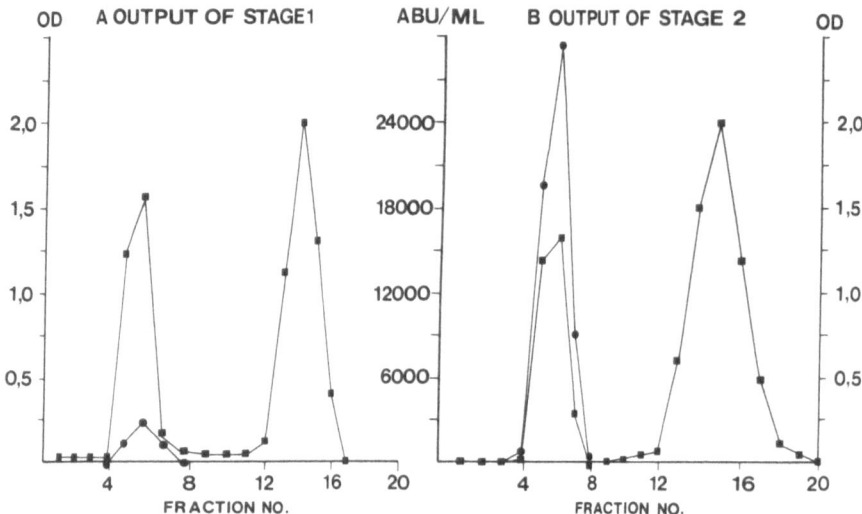

Figure 2

Preparation of Hemagglutinin from Purified Influenza Virus Particles

The purified virus particles were treated with bromelain first at 4°C for 2 hr to release neuraminidase (Stage 1) and then at 35°C for 2 hr to release hemagglutinin (Stage 2). The supernatants from each stage were filtered through a column of Sephadex G100 Superfine (1.6 x 24 cm) to separate either (A) neuraminidase or (B) hemagglutinin from bromelain. Uvicord I absorbance (O.D), ■———■ ; antibody blocking activity, ●———●

(Brand and Skehel, 1972; Skehel and Waterfield, 1975). Low levels (up to 7%) of the uncleaved precursor (HA) were found in all hemagglutinin preparations.

About 75 to 90% of the neuraminidase was removed in Stage 1 while the remainder was probably degraded in Stage 2 since no contaminating protein was present at detectable levels. Semi-cores showed no loss of hemagglutinating activity while cores showed a 90% reduction. The final yield of pure hemagglutinin ranged from 50 to 80% of the expected total calculated from Reimer's estimate of 4.2×10^{-6} gm protein per virus particle (Reimer *et al.*, 1966) and an assumption of 30-35% of protein as hemagglutinin (Schulze, 1973).

Separation of the Hemagglutinin Subunits

Molecular exclusion chromatography of hemagglutinin under reducing conditions or of CM-hemagglutinin on a column of Sepharose 6B or Bio-gel P150 in 6 M guanidine hydrochloride completely separated heavy and light subunits.

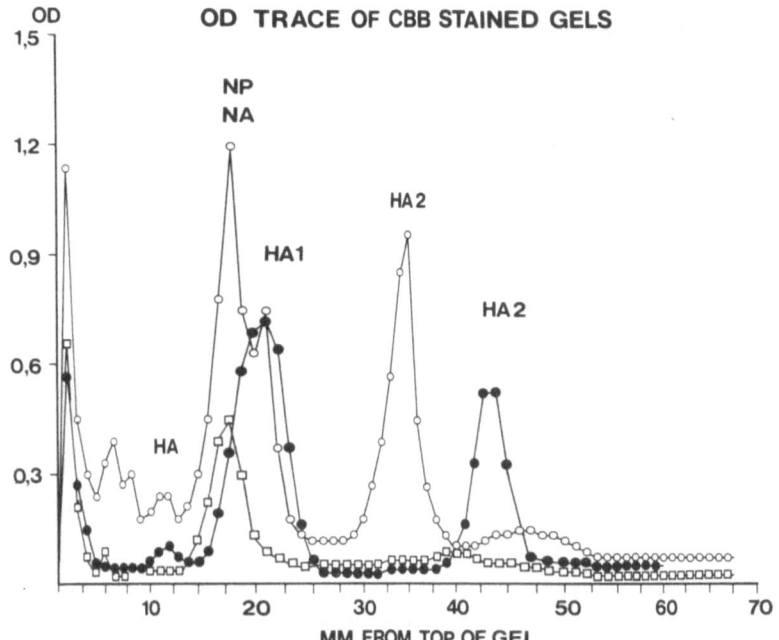

Figure 3

SDS-Polyacrylamide Gel Electrophoresis of Proteins from Purified Influenza Virus

Samples of purified virus and the bromelain-solubilized output fractions from Stages 1 and 2 of Figure 2 were treated with 2% SDS, 5% 2-mercaptoethanol for 2 min at 100°C and electro-phoresed on 10% polyacrylamide slab gels. Viral proteins were stained with Coomassie Brilliant Blue R250 (CBB) and the gels scanned at 570 nm.

Whole virus, o——o, neuraminidase (excluded peak of Stage 1), □——□, hemagglutinin (excluded peak of Stage 2), ●——●, HA, uncleaved precursor hemagglutinin; NP, nucleoprotein; NA, neuraminidase; HA$_1$, larger hemagglutinin subunit; HA$_2$, smaller hemagglutinin subunit; MP, matrix protein.

The polyacrylamide gel, Bio-gel P150 was preferred, since large amounts of degraded, interfering carbohydrate contaminated preparations from Sepharose 6B had been reported (Terhorst *et al.*, 1976).

Figure 4a shows the elution profile of NT60 CM-hemagglutinin. An identical profile was obtained for strain 29C. Only two peaks were revealed. Fractions were taken as indicated, dialyzed extensively to remove salts and analyzed.

SDS-Polyacrylamide Gel Electrophoresis

When unfractionated hemagglutinin preparations were analyzed by discontinu-ous electrophoresis on SDS-10% polyacrylamide gels under reducing conditions,

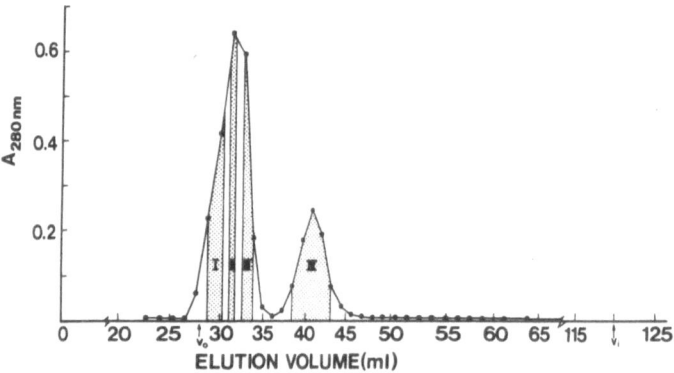

Figure 4a

Molecular Exclusion Chromatography of the Isolated Hemagglutinin from A3/NT60 on Bio-Gel P150

CM-hemagglutinin (**4 mg**) was applied to a column of Bio-Gel P150 (1.6 x 65 cm) and eluted with 6 M guanidine hydrochloride containing 0.05 M sodium acetate, 1 mM dithiothreitol, pH 5.0 to separate the larger (HA$_1$) and smaller (HA$_2$) subunits. Flow rate 2.4 ml/hr; fraction size 1.2 ml. Fractions analyzed are indicated by Roman numerals.

three protein bands could be detected (Figure 3): a minor one, HA, representing the uncleaved precursor hemagglutinin of 79,000 daltons, and two major ones, HA$_1$ and HA$_2$, representing the large and small subunits of 54,100 and 24,300 daltons respectively. The relative amount of HA was 5.8%, of HA$_1$ was 62.8% and of HA$_2$ was 31.4% when based on the absorbance value of Coomassie Blue stained bands at 570 nm.

The leading fraction (I) from the chromatographic column (Figure 4b) contained HA and some HA$_1$. Fraction II consisted of HA$_1$ with only a trace of HA (not shown). Fraction III was entirely HA$_1$, while Fraction IV was the small subunit, HA$_2$. The molecular weights of HA$_1$ and HA$_2$ were 53,700 and 24,200 respectively. These apparent molecular weights were overestimations because of the anomalous behavior of glycoproteins in SDS-polyacrylamide gels (Segrest and Jackson, 1972). By using polyacrylamide gels of increasing concentrations, a closer value to the true molecular weight can be obtained (Segrest and Jackson, 1972; Ward and Dopheide, 1976). In this way, a molecular weight of about 46,000 was obtained for HA$_1$ and 22,000 for HA$_2$. Moreover, molecular exclusion chromatography in 6 M guanidine hydrochloride suggested a molecular weight of 46,000 for HA$_1$ and 22,500 for HA$_2$. The value for HA$_1$ is in agreement with that of another Hong Kong variant, A/Memphis/102/72 (Moss and Hamilton, 1974) whereas that for HA$_2$ is somewhat lower,

OD TRACE OF CBB STAINED GELS

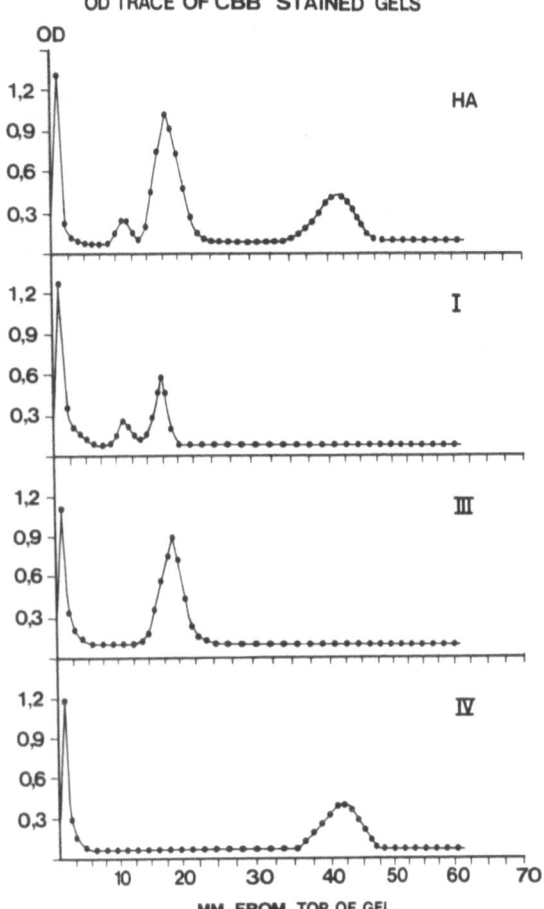

Figure 4b

SDS-polyacrylamide gel electrophoresis of whole hemagglutinin (HA) and fractions I, III and IV obtained after gel chromatography of isolated hemagglutinin from A3/NT60 in 6 M guanidine hydrochloride (see Figure 4a). The electrophoresis was carried out as described in Figure 3.

owing to the loss of a membrane bound fragment during bromelain digestion of the viral coat (Brand and Skehel, 1972; Skehel and Waterfield, 1975). Published data suggest that HA_1 contains about 24% carbohydrates, whereas HA_2 contains about 5% (Ward and Dopheide, 1976). Therefore the molecular weight of the protein moiety of HA_1 most likely lies between 35,000 and 41,000, (say 38,000) and of HA_2 between 21,000 and 23,000 (say 22,000).

Amino Acid Compositions

Table 1 presents amino acid compositions of unfractionated hemagglutinin (HA) large (HA$_1$) and small (HA$_2$) subunits from the influenza virus strain NT60. In the absence of true molecular weights, the tentative values of 38,000, 22,000 and 60,000 daltons respectively, for the protein moieties of HA$_1$, HA$_2$ and HA, have been used to derive the number of amino acid residues per mole. The internal consistency of the amino acid compositions of unfractionated HA and the sum of HA$_1$ and HA$_2$ (assuming a molecular ration of 1:1), together with SDS-polyacrylamide gel analysis, NH$_2$-terminal sequence analysis and tryptic peptide mapping, suggest that no significant contamination of the hemagglutinin preparation occurs.

NH$_2$-Terminal Amino Acid Sequences

The NH$_2$-terminal amino acids in the hemagglutinin of NT60 were analyzed by SDS-dansyl-Edman procedure. Hydrolysis of the dansylated protein with either 6 M HCl or Pronase (Tamura *et al.*, 1973; Moss and Hamilton, 1974) revealed only glycine as the NH$_2$-terminal end group in whole HA. A minimum of two end groups were expected, one for each subunit. No NH$_2$-terminal amino acid was detected in HA$_1$, so it must be concluded that this subunit is blocked. The nature of the blocking group is unknown. Glycine was the only detectable end group in HA$_2$. Since only one NH$_2$-terminal end group was revealed in HA it seems likely that no random proteolysis of the hemagglutinin occurs during bromelain treatment. The bromelain apparently acts at a cleavage site near the carboxyl terminal end of the HA$_2$ subunit (Skehel and Waterfield, 1975; Bucher *et al.*, 1976).

Partial NH$_2$-terminal sequences of NT60 and 29C hemagglutinins give the results shown in Table 2. HA$_1$ was blocked in both strains. Identical sequences were obtained in both HA$_2$ subunits, which corresponded with other influenza A virus strains (Skehel and Waterfield, 1975; Bucher *et al.*, 1976).

Peptide Maps of Hemagglutinin

Fluorescent dansyl-peptide mapping by two-dimensional thin layer chromatography on silica gel G was the chosen method since only small amounts of protein (15-65 μg) were required. This facilitated comparison of hemagglutinins available in only nanomole amounts. The method has been effectively used on a nanomole scale both in the comparative analysis of related proteins and in the partial determination of the primary structure of proteins (Zanetta *et al.*, 1970; Moss and Hamilton, 1974; Schmer and Kreil, 1967; Spivak *et al.*, 1971). Preliminary experiments with reference proteins such as bovine serum albumin, hen

Table 1

Amino Acid Compositions of Unfractionated Hemagglutinin (HA), Heavy Subunit (HA$_1$) and Light Subunit (HA$_2$) from the Influenza Virus Strain NT60

(Values are expressed as residues per 100 residues (i) and residues per mole protein (ii))

Amino Acid	HA$_1$ (i)	HA$_1$ (ii) 38,000 daltons	HA$_2$ (i)	HA$_2$ (ii) 22,000 daltons	HA (i)	HA (ii) 60,000 daltons	HA$_1$ + HA$_2$ (ii)
LYS	4.82	16.3	6.55	12.8	5.46	29.1	29.1
HIS	1.74	5.9	2.68	5.2	2.14	11.4	11.1
ARG	5.87	19.8	4.91	9.6	5.53	29.5	29.4
SCM-CYS	2.08	7.0	1.49	2.9	1.84	9.8	9.9
ASP	13.18	44.5	14.54	28.5	13.59	72.4	73.0
THR*	7.82	26.4	4.62	9.1	6.72	35.8	35.5
SER*	8.26	27.9	4.67	9.2	7.23	38.6	37.1
GLU	8.90	30.1	16.90	33.1	10.74	57.2	63.2
PRO	5.47	18.5	0.94	1.8	4.17	22.2	20.3
GLY	8.50	28.7	9.78	19.2	9.26	49.4	47.9
ALA	5.57	18.8	6.55	12.8	6.08	32.4	31.6
VAL	6.13	20.7	3.42	6.7	5.35	28.5	27.4
MET	1.78	6.0	1.29	2.5	1.52	8.1	8.5
ILE	6.45	21.8	7.30	14.3	6.38	34.0	36.1
LEU	7.26	24.6	6.95	13.6	7.20	38.4	38.2
TYR	2.96	10.0	3.13	6.1	3.13	16.7	16.1
PHE	3.23	10.9	4.22	8.3	3.58	19.1	19.2
TRP**	N.D.		N.D.		N.D.		

* Values extrapolated to zero time to correct for hydrolytic losses   ** Tryptophan was not determined

Table 2

NH$_2$-Terminal Amino Acid Sequences of Hemagglutinin Subunits

Virus Strain	HA$_1$	HA$_2$
NT60	Blocked	GLY–LEU–PHE–
29C	Blocked	GLY–LEU–PHE–

egg lysozyme and chicken globins established that 90% or more of the expected peptides could be accounted for on the maps.

Carboxamidomethylated or carboxymethylated hemagglutinin was digested with trypsin and the resultant peptides dansylated, then 'fingerprinted'. Figures 5-7 represent diagrammatically the fluorescent dansyl-peptide maps so obtained.

Preliminary fingerprinting studies with carboxamidomethyl NT60 hemagglutinin from several independent experiments using replicate samples indicated the presence of approximately 61 diagnostic spots and 7 very faint but reproducible spots. Although the fingerprints were virtually identical, especially when run in parallel, only co-chromatography of different dansylated tryptic digests and consequent comigration of the peptides permitted a confident interpretation of identity. No peptides from self-digestion of trypsin were evident in control runs omitting hemagglutinin.

Figure 5 shows comparative peptide maps of carboxamidomethylated hemagglutinins for the hierarchic series NT60, 375/17, 29C and 142/6. All maps reveal notably similar patterns, with the exception of apparently one variable peptide (indicated by the arrows). Co-chromatography of the tryptic peptides from various combinations of members of the hierarchic series established the aberrant nature of the variable peptide. Resolution of this peptide was not always clear-cut, however. No other peptides seemed to manifest this variable property.

Since carboxamidomethyl-cysteine residues might be subject to hydrolysis by trypsin (Means and Feeney, 1975) leading to gratuitous peptides, further work was undertaken with the carboxymethyl derivative. Figure 6 depicts comparative peptide maps of carboxymethylated hemagglutinins from the strains NT60, 375/17, 29C, and 30C. The solvent systems used in preparing these maps also differed in that they were rendered 5 mM in 2-mercaptoethanol to protect methionine and help stabilize the fluorescence (Tamura *et al.*, 1973). These maps are fundamentally similar to those derived from carboxamidomethylated HA (Figure 5). However, some peptides had obviously different mobilities while other peptides seen in Figure 5 were absent or not well resolved in Figure 6. It

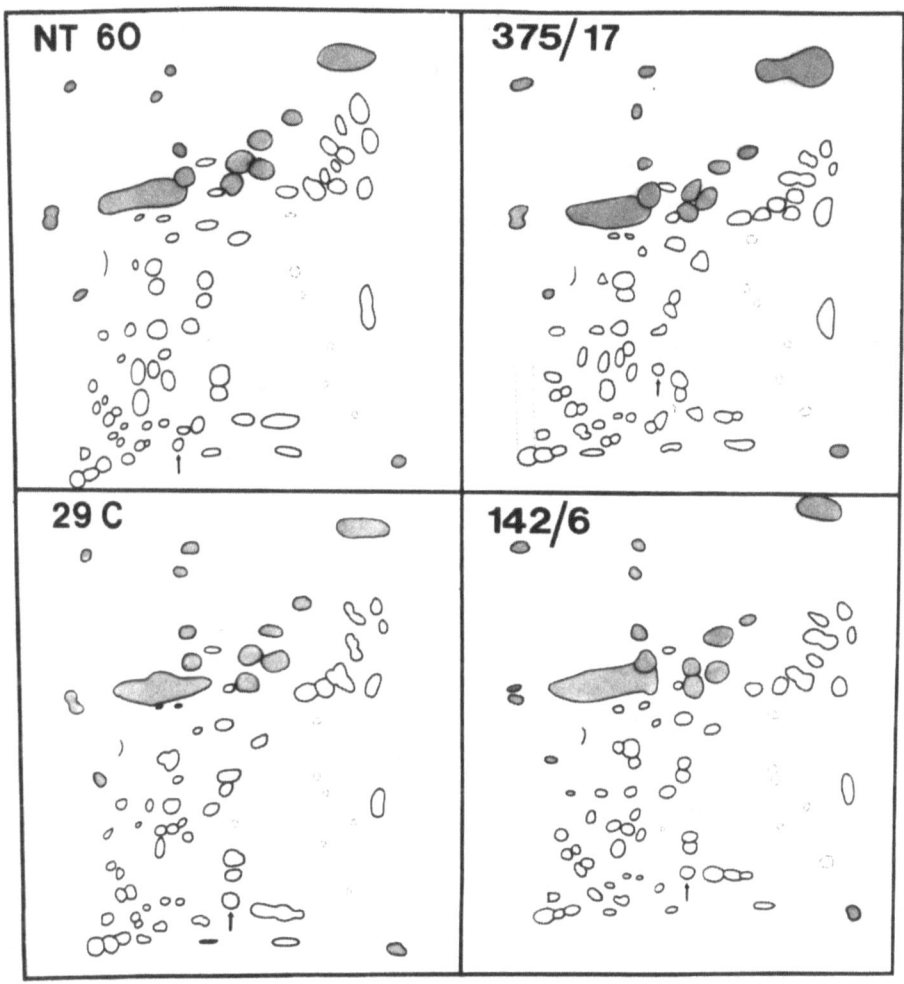

Figure 5

Tracings of Tryptic Fingerprints of Fluorescent Dansyl-Peptides Derived from Hemagglutinins of the Hierarchic Antigenic Mutants NT60, 375/17, 29C and 142/6

Hemagglutinin was reduced and carboxamidomethylated, digested with trypsin-TPCK and dansylated. The dansyl-peptides (from 1 nmole of hemagglutinin) were separated by two-dimensional chromatography at 20°C on silica gel G thin-layer plates (20 cm x 20 cm). Each dimension is indicated by a Roman numeral. Chromatography in the first dimension (methyl acetate-isopropanol-25% ammonia; 9:6:4, by vol.) was for 1.5 hr followed by development in the second dimension (isobutanol-acetic acid-water; 15:4:2, by vol.) for 3.5 hr. The shaded areas indicate spots resulting from the reagents used. Peptides apparently different are indicated by arrows.

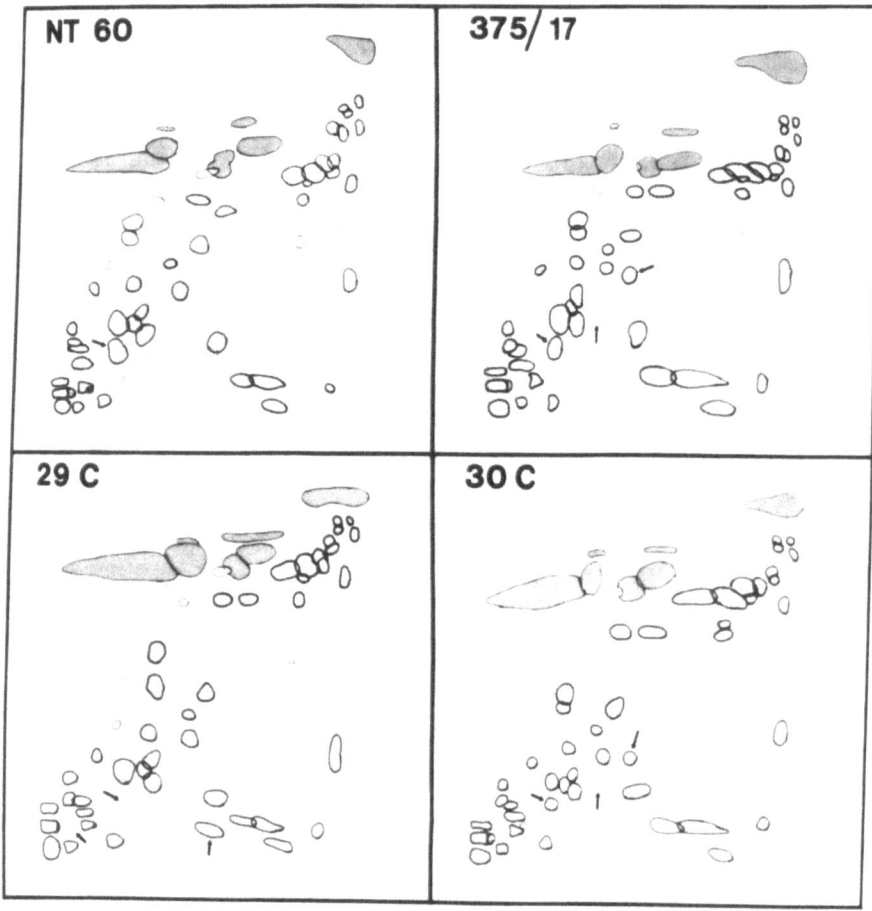

Figure 6

Tracings of Tryptic Fingerprints of Fluorescent Dansyl-Peptides Derived from Hemagglutinins of the Antigenic Mutants NT60, 375/17, 29C and 30C

The same conditions as described in Figure 5 were used except that the hemagglutinins were reduced and carboxymethylated and the solvents for chromatography were rendered 5 mM in 2-mercaptoethanol. Peptides apparently different are indicated by arrows.

was clear from comparisons within the set of CM-hemagglutinins (Figure 6) that one or two peptides (indicated by the arrows) were variable. Once again, co-chromatography of various combinations of the mutant virus strains confirmed the aberrant nature of these peptides. These maps suggested that there were approximately 50 diagnostic spots and 8 very faint, reproducible spots. There-fore, from a consideration of Figures 5 and 6 there seems to be a minimum of

50 dansyl-peptides, excluding faintly fluorescent spots, ranging to 68 when all spots are counted.

Based on the lysine plus arginine content of the hemagglutinin (Table 1), the expected maximum number of tryptic peptides for HA would be 60, provided the subunits are totally different and complete resolution of peptides is effected. HA_1 and HA_2 should yield 37 and 24 peptides respectively. However, since the intensity of fluorescence is not proportional to the amount of peptide per spot, it is difficult to assign exact numbers of peptides from fluorescent fingerprints (Zanetta *et al.*, 1970; Vandekerckhove and van Montagu, 1974; Fey and Hirt, 1974).

In order to simplify the complex patterns of the fingerprints and to determine which subunit contained the variable peptide(s), the carboxymethylated HA_1 and HA_2 subunits from NT60 and 29C were subjected to fingerprint analysis (Figure 7).

HA_1 from both NT60 and 29C showed 34-40 fluorescent dansyl-peptide spots, while HA_2 showed 22-28, which are within the tentative theoretical ranges. Therefore, it seems likely that most, if not all, of the tryptic peptides are represented by this fluorescent fingerprinting technique. Maps of HA_2 were identical, whereas those of HA_1 showed one major and one minor spot to be variable as indicated by the arrows. Leucine was the NH_2-terminal amino acid in the major variable spots. Qualitative analysis of the variable major and minor spots indicated a complex mixture of amino acids with no obvious differences. The main amino acids present were glycine, proline, valine, leucine, phenylalanine, bis-lysine with lesser amounts of isoleucine, bis-tyrosine, serine and some methionine and arginine. The presence in the peptides of tyrosine and methionine, which can have differing reactivities or can be oxidized, may in part account for the occurence of the minor variable spot. The appearance of both lysine and arginine suggests either partial cleavage of the peptide by trypsin or the presence of two peptides. No firm conclusions can be drawn from these incomplete results until more exacting quantitative analyses have been undertaken.

Radioautography of the hemagglutinin subunits from NT60 and 29C showed 8 cysteinyl-peptides in HA_1 (Figure 7). This number agreed with the number predicted from the CM-cysteine content (Table 1). The variable spots were not associated with these cysteinyl peptides. HA_2 on the other hand, had only two cysteinyl peptides, which was less than the expected number. Two cysteine residues in a common peptide may account for this observation.

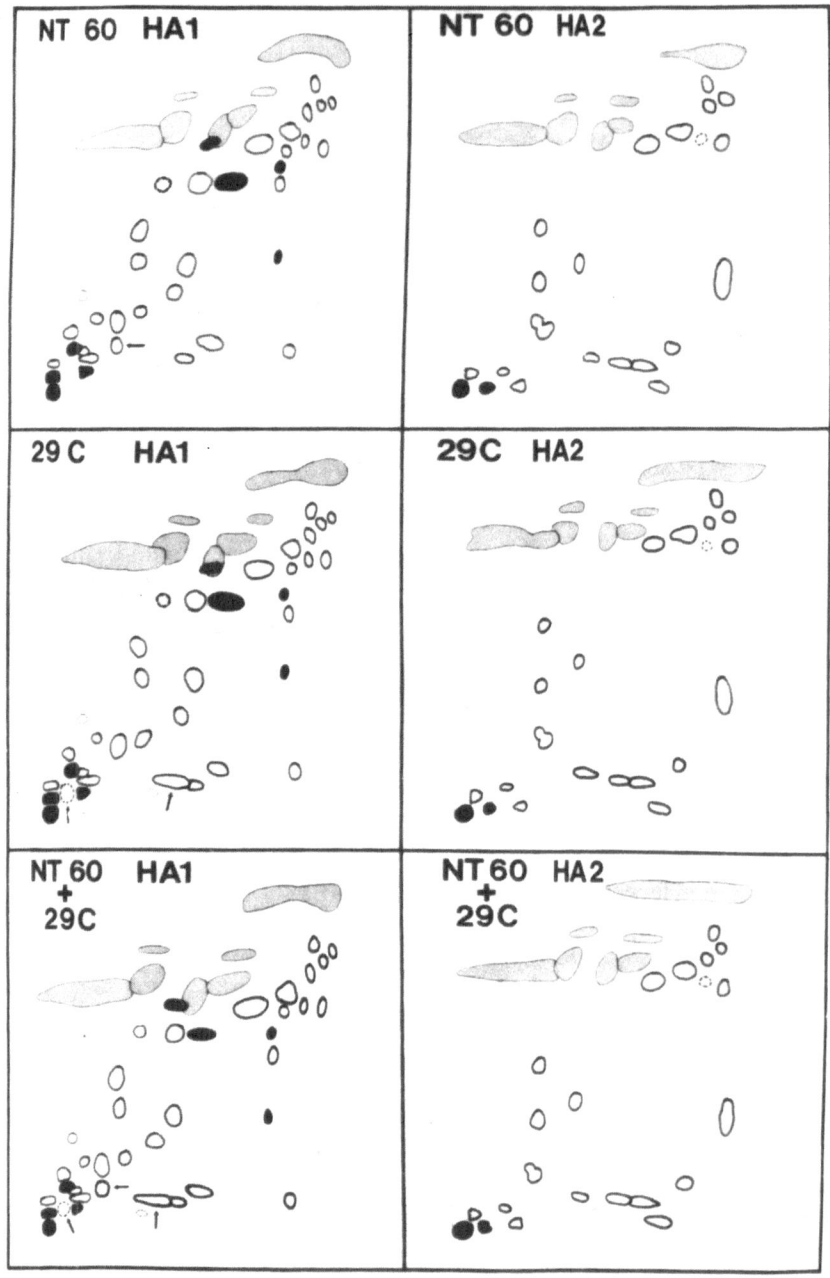

Figure 7

Tracings of Tryptic Fingerprints of Fluorescent Dansyl-Peptides Derived from the
Hemagglutinin Subunits, HA_1 and HA_2, of Virus Strains NT60 and 29C

The same conditions as described in Figure 6 were used. The corresponding subunits from both strains were also subjected to co-chromatography. Peptides apparently different are indicated by the arrows. The solid areas indicate spots containing ^{14}C-carboxymethyl-cysteine.

Discussion

It is recognized that changes in the primary structure of both hemagglutinin and neuraminidase accompany the observed serological variability of influenza viruses (Laver and Webster, 1968, 1971, 1973; Webster and Laver, 1971; Laver et al., 1974; Laver, 1973; Kendal and Eckert, 1972; Kendal and Kiley, 1973). However, chemical studies on the mechanism of antigenic variation can be complicated by many factors. For example, it has been common practice to disrupt the virus with detergents during protein isolation. Such treatment may denature the proteins rendering them unsuitable for serological tests, and traces of firmly bound detergent could interfere with enzymic and chemical analysis. Conventional peptide mapping (Ingram, 1958; Bennett, 1967; Laver, 1969), whilst being a powerful tool in protein structural studies, cannot effectively resolve electrophoretically neutral peptides. Moreover, in the case of influenza virus hemagglutinin, up to 60% of the tryptic peptides, as insoluble 'core' peptides, may be overlooked (Laver and Webster, 1968,1971,1973; Webster and Laver, 1971; Laver et al., 1974; Laver, 1964,1973). To date, the analysis of viral strains has not discriminated between adsorptive, adaptive and gratuitous mutations in the hemagglutinin molecule (Fazekas de St. Groth, 1977), and those due to antigenic mutation. While the peptides analyzed represent an arbitrary fraction of the total, and the genetic lineage of the viruses is generally unknown, our understanding of the mechanism of antigenic variation has no molecular basis.

For these reasons we sought to use an isogenic series of mutants with changes restricted to the antigenic region of the hemagglutinin molecule. Such a series of antigenic mutants has been described previously (Fazekas de St. Groth, 1975, 1977; Fazekas de St. Groth and Hannoun, 1973). We also sought to isolate antigenically intact hemagglutinin for the series capable of being analyzed by a fingerprinting method resolving most if not all of the tryptic peptides.

This report confirms that soluble, antigenically active hemagglutinin could be released from influenza virions by bromelain treatment (Brand and Skehel, 1972; Skehel and Waterfield, 1975). The hemagglutinin was conveniently separated from the neuraminidase by the sequential two-stage temperature-dependent process described. The final product obtained by molecular exclusion chromatography was apparently free of contamination as judged by SDS-polyacrylamide gel electrophoresis, NH$_2$-terminal amino acid analysis, amino acid composition and tryptic peptide mapping. The hemagglutinin isolated by this proteolytic method did not seem to differ significantly in size from detergent released hemagglutinin except that HA_2, the membrane associated subunit, was slightly smaller, in agreement with earlier reports (Brand and Skehel, 1972; Skehel and Waterfield, 1975). The partial NH_2-terminal sequence data of HA_2 coincided with the corresponding subunits from other influenza virus strains thereby confirming that host (chick) proteases cleave the precursor hemagglutinin molecule at a common point (Tamura *et al.*, 1973; Bucher *et al.*, 1976). The NH_2-terminal of HA_1 is apparently blocked.

The remarkable similarity in the fingerprints of hemagglutinins obtained from the different viral strains and the close agreement of the number of fluorescent spots with the expected number of peptides makes it likely that virtually all of the tryptic peptides are represented. The comparative fingerprints allow is to conclude that, with the exception of one or two variable peptides, the primary structures of the mutant hemagglutinins are identical. The limited variation in the primary structure of the hemagglutinin, therefore, is associated with the observed antigenic changes. The comparative fingerprint data are consistent with a minimal number of chemical changes occurring in the hemagglutinin molecule, confined to the larger subunit HA_1. Earlier studies by others have shown that peptide maps of HA_1 exhibit wider variability than those of HA_2 (Laver and Webster, 1968,1971,1973; Webster and Laver, 1971; Laver *et al.*, 1974; Laver, 1973), and that the antigenicity of hemagglutinin is elicited by HA_1 rather than HA_2 (Brand and Skehel, 1972; Eckert, 1973; Moss and Underwood unpublished data).

The structural changes in HA_1 are interpreted as resulting from mutations in the polypeptide chain. Whether the variable peptides are part of the antigenic determinants *per se*, or occupy some other part of the molecule which, nevertheless, profoundly affects the conformation of the antigenic region requires elucidation. However, since the virus strains have been selected on the basis of antigenic mutations it is tempting to suggest that the variable peptides are not only correlated with mutational changes, but form part of the antigenic determinant. A formal proof requires the demonstration of the variable peptides in antigenically active fragments.

REFERENCES

BENNETT, J. C. (1967) Methods in Enzymology, Vol. XI, 330-339.

BRAND, C. M. and SKEHEL, J. J. (1976) Nature New Biol. *238*, 145-147.

BUCHER, D. J., LI, S. S-L., KEHOE, J. M. and KILBOURNE, E. D. (1976) Proc. Nat. Acad. Sci. USA. *73*, 238-242.

ECKERT, E. A. (1973) J. Virol, *11*, 183-192.

FAZEKAS DE ST. GROTH, S. (1952) J. Hyg. Camb. *50*, 471-490.

FAZEKAS DE ST. GROTH, S. (1969a) J. Immunol. *103*, 1107-1115.

FAZEKAS DE ST. GROTH, S. (1969b) Bull. WHO *41*, 651-657.

FAZEKAS DE ST. GROTH, S. (1970) Arch. Environ. Health *21*, 293-303.

FAZEKAS DE ST. GROTH, S. (1975) in 'Negative Strand Viruses', (Mahy, B. W. J. and Barry, R. D., eds.) Academic Press. London. Vol.2, 741-754.

FAZEKAS DE ST. GROTH, S. (1977) this volume.

FAZEKAS DE ST. GROTH, S. and CAIRNS, H. J. F. (1952) J. Immunol. *69*, 173.

FAZEKAS DE ST. GROTH, S. and FORSTER, H. (1973) Annual Report of the Basel Institute for Immunology, pp. 99.

FAZEKAS DE ST. GROTH, S. and GRAHAM, D. M. (1955) Brit. J. Exp. Path. *35*, 60-74.

FAZEKAS DE ST. GROTH, S. and HANNOUN, C. (1973) Compte Rendu Acad. Sci. Paris, *276*, 1917-1920 (series D)

FEY, G. and HIRT, B. (1974) Cold Spring Harbor Symp. Quant. Biol. *39*, 235-241.

FRANCIS, T. and SHOPE, R. E. (1936) J. Exp. Med. *63*, 645-653.

GREEN, R. W. and BOLOGNESI, D. P. (1974) Anal Biochem. *57*, 108-117.

GROS, C. (1967) Bull. Soc. Chimi. France, *10*, 3952-3954.

INGRAM, V. M. (1958) Biochim. Biophys. Acta *28*, 539.

KAPITANY, R. A. and ZEBROWSKI, E. J. (1973) Anal Biochem. *56*, 361-369.

KENDAL, A. P. and ECKERT, E. A. (1972) Biochim. Biophys. Acta *258*, 484-495.

KENDAL, A. P. and KILEY, M. P. (1973) J. Virol. *12*, 1482-1490.

LAEMMLI, U. K. (1970) Nature *227*, 680-685.

LAVER, W. G. (1964) J. Mol. Biol. *9*, 109-124.

LAVER, W. G. (1969) in 'Fundamental Techniques in Virology' (Habel, K.and Salzman, N. eds.) Academic Press, N.Y. 371-378.

LAVER, W. G. (1973) in 'Advances in Virus Research' (Lauffer, M. A., Bang, F. B., Maramorasch, K. and Smith, K. M., eds.) Academic Press, N.Y., *18*, 57-103.

LAVER, W. G., DOWNIE, J. C. and WEBSTER, R. G. (1974) Virology *59*, 230-244.

LAVER, W. G. and WEBSTER, R. G. (1968) Virology *34*, 193-202.

LAVER, W. G. and WEBSTER, R. G. (1971) Virology *48*, 445-455.

LAVER, W. G. and WEBSTER, R. G. (1973) Virology *51*, 383-391.

LAYNE, E. (1957) Methods in Enzymology, Vol. III, 447-454.

MAGILL, T. P. and FRANCIS, T. (1936) Proc. Soc. Exp. Biol. Med. *35*, 463-466.

MARGOLIS, J. and KENRICK, K. G. (1968) Anal. Biochem. *25*, 347-362.

MEANS, G. E. and FEENEY, R. E. (1975) Chemical Modification of Proteins. Holden-Day Inc., San Francisco.

MOSS, B. A. (1977) Methods in Immunology. Academic Press, Manuscript in preparation.

MOSS, B. A. and HAMILTON, E. A. (1974) Biochim. Biophys. Acta *371*, 379-391.

REIMER, C. B., BAKER, R. S., NEULIN, T. W. and HAVENS, M. L. (1966) Science *152*, 1503-1504.

SCHMER, G. and KREIL, G. (1967) J. Chromatog. *28*, 458-461.

SCHULZE, I. T. (1973) Adv. Virus Res. *18*, 1-55.

SEGREST, J. P. and JACKSON, R. L. (1972) Methods in Enzymology, Vol. XXVIII, 54-63.

SKEHEL, J. J. and WATERFIELD, M. D. (1975) Proc. Nat. Acad. Sci. USA. *72*, 93-97.

SMORODINTSEFF, A. A., DROBYSHEVSKAYA, A. I. and SHISHKINA, O. I. (1936) Lancet *2*, 1383-1385.

SPIVAK, V. A., LEVJANT, S. P., KATRUKHA, S. P. and VARSHAVSKY, J. M. (1971) Anal. Biochem. *44*, 503-518.

STONE, J. D. (1949) Aust. J. Exp. Biol. *27*, 337-352.

TAMURA, Z., NAKAJIMA, T., NAKAYAMA, T., PISANO, J. J. and UDENFRIEND, S. (1973) Anal. Biochem. *52*, 595-606.

TERHORST, C. PARHAM, P., MANN, D. L. and STROMINGER, J. L. (1976) Proc. Nat. Acad. Sci. USA. *73*, 910-914.

VANDEKERCKHOVE, J. and VAN MONTAGU, M. (1974) Eur. J. Biochem. *44*, 279-288.

WARD, C. W. and DOPHEIDE, T. A. A. (1976) FEBS Letters *65*, 365-368.

WEBSTER, R. G. and LAVER, W. G. (1971) Progr. Med. Virol. *13*, 271-338.

WEINER, A. M., PLATT, T. and WEBER, K. (1972) J. Biol. Chem. *247*, 3242-3251.

ZANETTA, J. P. VINCENDON, G., MANDEL, P. and GOMBOS, G. (1970) J. Chromatog. *51*, 441-458.

STRUCTURAL STUDIES OF THE HEMAGGLUTININ OF THE ASIAN INFLUENZA VIRUS JAPAN/305/57 - BELLAMY/42 (H2N1).CYANOGEN BROMIDE CLEAVAGE OF THE LARGER POLYPEPTIDE CHAIN HA$_1$

M. D. Waterfield, J. J. Skehel, Y. Nakashima, A. Gurnett, and T. Bilham

Summary

A structural study of the hemagglutinin from the influenza virus variant Japan/305/57 - Bellamy/42 (H2N1) is described. The two disulfide bonded glycopolypeptide chains (BHA$_1$ and BHA$_2$ were separated from the hemagglutinin which had been released from virus with stem Bromelain (EC 3.4.22.4). The larger glycopolypeptide BHA$_1$ contained 25% carbohydrate composed of fucose, mannose, galactose and N-acetyl glucosamine in the ratio (1:3: 3.2:5.4), linked through asparagine side chains to a polypeptide chain of approximately 340 amino acids. Cyanogen bromide (CNBr) cleavage of BHA$_1$ is described. Seven CNBr fragments have been purified and their order partially determined by sequence analysis of overlapping protease generated peptides. Three CNBr peptides are glycosylated and three peptides contain cysteine residues. The implications of this study on knowledge of the hemagglutinin structure and function is discussed.

Introduction

The envelope of influenza virus contains 2 glycoproteins – the hemagglutinin and the neuraminidase. The hemagglutinin is involved in interaction with the cell during infection and is the component against which neutralizing antibodies are directed (Schulze, 1973; Laver, 1973). To study antigenic variation, and to define the interactions of glycoproteins with lipid membranes, the complete primary structure of the hemagglutinin (HA) from an Asian strain of virus is being determined. The HA is in the major envelope protein of the virus and forms 30% of the virus protein (Schulze, 1973; Laver, 1973). HA is probably a trimer on the virus having subunits with apparent molecular weights of 75-80,000 on SDS polyacrylamide gels (Wiley *et al.*, 1977). Each subunit consists of 2 disulfide bonded polypeptide chains of apparent molecular weights 55-58,000 (HA$_1$) and 25-30,000 (HA$_2$) (Laver, 1971; Lazarowitz *et al.*, 1971; Skehel and Waterfield, 1975). The carboxyl terminus of HA$_2$ is associated with the virus membrane and the biosynthetic amino terminus is on HA_1 (Skehel and Waterfield, 1975). Proteolytic cleavage of the single polypeptide chain bio-synthetic precursor forms the 2 component chains HA_1 and HA_2. Virus with cleaved HA is more infectious than virus containing uncleaved precursor HA (Klenk et al., 1972, 1975; Hay, 1974). This paper describes the characterization of the cyanogen bromide cleavage products of the larger polypeptide chain HA_1. A similar study of the smaller chain HA_2 is described in the accompanying paper (McCauley et al., 1977). These results form a basis for the elucidation of the primary structure of the HA.

Methods

Virus

Viruses were grown in the allantoic cavity of 10-day-old embryonated eggs. Japan/305/57 - Bellamy/42 (H2N1) was a recombinant isolated at the World Influenza Centre, London. Viruses were concentrated and purified as previous-ly described (Skehel and Schild, 1971).

Hemagglutinin Isolation

a. Virus particles were disrupted in 2% (w/v) sodium dodecyl sulfate at 20^0 and the proteins separated by electrophoresis on Celogel (Chemetron, Milan) as supporting medium.
b. Virus particles were digested with stem Bromelain (Sigma EC 3.4.22.4) and the released hemagglutinin purified by sucrose density gradient centrifugation.

Separation of Hemagglutinin Polypeptide Chains

a. The two chains of the hemagglutinin from detergent disrupted virus were separated by guanidine HCl gradients (Laver, 1971) or by chromatography on Sephadex G200 (Pharmacia) in 6 M urea containing 0.2 M formic acid following full reduction and alkylation of disulfide groups with iodoacet-amide (Skehel and Waterfield, 1975).
b. The two chains of the Bromelain released hemagglutinin were separated on Sephadex G100 following full reduction and alkylation (Skehel and Waterfield, 1975).

Sequence Analysis

Amino acid analyses were preformed on a Durrum D500 amino acid analyser following 24 hr hydrolysis of samples in 6NHCl containing 3 μM butane dithiol and 0.1% phenol using the procedures of Smyth *et al.* (1963). Sequence analysis was carried out using either (a) the micro dansyl Edman technique of Hartley (1970) or (b) the automatic liquid phase Sequencer (Beckman 890C) employing a dilute quadrol program (Brauer *et al.*, 1975). PTH amino acids were analyzed by (a) gas liquid chromatography using the method of Pisano and Bronzert (1969). (b) High pressure liquid chromatography using a μ-bondapak C^{18} reversed phase column 0.4 x 20 cm (Walters Assoc., Mass. USA.) or (c) by amino acid analysis following back hydrolysis (Smithies *et al.*, 1971). Cysteine residues were located by monitoring radioactivity in ^{14}C-carboxamidomethyl cysteine during sequence analysis. Cyanogen bromide cleavage was by the method of Gross and Witkop (1961). Carbohydrate analyses were performed by gas liquid chromatography of tri-methyl silylated derivatives by a modification of the method of Lane *et al.* (1972). Peptides were fractionated on columns of either SP or QAE Sephadex (Pharmacia) Chromobeads P (Technicon) or DAX2 (Durrum) using volatile buffers. In most cases a portion of the column effluent was monitored for ninhydrin positive material by the procedure of Herman and Vanaman (1975). Peptide separations on Sephadex G50 in ammonia-propan-1-ol were monitored with a UVICORD III (LKB) at 206 nm. Paper electrophoresis was by the method of Katz *et al.* (1959).

Results

The HA has been isolated from the virus by 2 different procedures (a) disruption of the virus in SDS followed by electrophoresis on cellulose acetate strips or (b) by treatment of the virus with the protease Bromelain (EC 3.4.22.4). The HA isolated by both techniques consists of 2 disulfide bonded polypeptide chains, which may be separated by sieving on Sephadex columns under denaturing conditions following reduction and alkylation of disulfide bonds. The component chains of the HA from virus disrupted with SDS (HA_1 and HA_2) have been separated on Sephadex G200 using 6 M urea containing 0.2 M formic acid. Under these conditions HA_2, the smaller polypeptide, aggregates and is excluded from the column while HA_1 runs as a monomer. The component chains of the bromelain released HA (BHA_1 and BHA_2) have been separated on Sephadex G100 in urea and formic acid under which conditions both chains run as monomers (Skehel and Waterfield, 1975). The difference in aggregation properties of HA_2 and BHA_2 is probably due to the removal of the hydrophobic tail from the BHA_2 molecule during release of the HA spike from the virus by Bromelain digestion.

Amino acid analysis and carbohydrate analysis of HA_1 and BHA_1 showed that the glycopolypeptides were identical within the limits of the method. The present studies have all been performed with the glycopolypeptide BHA_1. The amino acid and carbohydrate analysis of BHA_1 is summarized in Table 1. The results are based on 338 amino acid residues which are derived from structural studies of the cyanogen bromide cleavage products described below. The total molecular weight of the glycopolypeptide which contains 24.4% carbohydrate is 50,000.

Table 1

Amino Acid and Carbohydrate Composition of the Large Polypeptide BHA_1 from the Hemagglutinin of Jap/305 - Bel/42 (H2N1) Influenza Virus

Residues/Mole Protein

Aspartic acid	35.9
Threonine	32.9
Serine	26.0
Glutamic acid	37.6
Proline	17.9
Glycine	29.8
Alanine	11.3
Valine	17.8
Methionine	5.4
Isoleucine	18.8
Leucine	30.4
Tyrosine	10.4
Phenylalanine	8.7
Histidine	10.3
Lysine	22.5
Arginine	13.2
Cysteine	9.6
Fucose	5.4
Mannose	16.2
Galactose	17.3
N-acetylglucosamine	29.1

Results are based on 338 amino acid residues excluding tryptophan

Cyanogen Bromide Cleavage

The BHA_1 glycopolypeptide was cleaved with cyanogen bromide in 70% formic acid for 18 hours (Smithies et al., 1971) and the digest lyophilized. Sequence

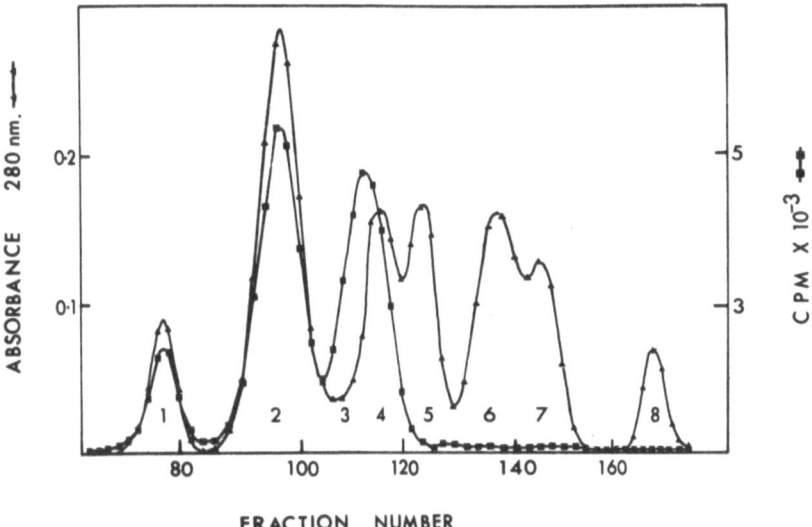

Figure 1

Fractionation of Cyanogen Bromide Cleavage Products of BHA$_1$

Peptides were separated on a 90 x 2.5 cm column of Sephadex G100 in 6 M urea containing
0.2 M formic acid. Absorbance at 280 mµ and radioactivity in [^{14}C] carboxamidomethyl
cysteine were measured on aliquots of each fraction. Numbers indicate the cyanogen bromide
peptides referred to in the text. Peptides 3 and 4 were subfractionated as shown in Figure 2.

analysis of the whole digest in the Beckman sequencer revealed six amino terminal residues (aspartic acid, glutamic acid, valine, leucine, lysine and tryptophan)
of which glutamic acid was present in 1.5 times the molar yield of the other
residues. The cyanogen bromide digest was dissolved in 6 M guanidine and incubated at 37°C for 2 hours to disrupt aggregates before fractionation on
Sephadex G100 in 6 M urea containing 0.2 M formic acid. The separation of
the peptides is shown in Figure 1. The location of cysteine containing peptides
was made by monitoring for the ^{14}C carboxamidomethyl cysteine residues introduced during full reduction and alkylation with ^{14}C iodoacetamide. Eight
distinct peptides were revealed by the separation of which 4 contained cysteine.
Peptide 3 showed a very low absorbence compared with the other peptides. All
peptides were desalted on G25 Sephadex in 0.25 M acetic acid and lyophilized.
Peptides 1 and 2 were further purified by rechromatography on G100 in 6 M
urea containing 0.2 M formic acid. Peptides 3 and 4 were fractionated by ion
exchange chromatography on SP-Sephadex in pyridine acetate buffers (Figure
2) and peptides 5, 6 and 7 were purified by chromatography on Sephadex G50

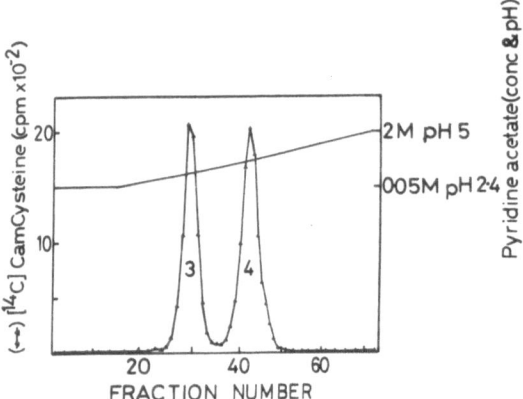

Figure 2

Separation of Cyanogen Bromide Peptides 3 and 4 on SP Sephadex

The peptides were applied to a 0.9 x 15 cm column of SP-Sephadex C-25 in 0.05 M pyridine acetate buffer pH 2.4. The column was developed with a linear gradient of pyridine acetate from 0.05 M pH 2.4 to 2.0 M pH 5. Aliquots of each fraction were monitored for radioactive [^{14}C] carboxamidomethyl cysteine.

in 0.25 M acetic acid. The amino acid compositions of the individual cyanogen bromide peptides are given in Table 2. The total amino acid composition of fragments 2-8 is very similar to the composition of the whole polypeptide (Table 1). Amino terminal sequence analysis (Table 3) showed that peptides 2-8 each had distinct sequences while peptide 1 had the same sequence as peptide 2. Analysis of the tryptic peptides of CNBr peptides 1, 2 and 4 isolated by ion exchange chromatography on columns showed that peptide 1 contained tryptic peptides which were present in the digests of peptides 2 and 4. The amino acid composition of peptide 1 was very similar to the sum of the compositions of peptides 2 and 4. This data suggested that peptide 1 was a partial cleavage product of peptides 2 and 4.

Sequence analysis of CNBr peptide 4 revealed an amino terminal sequence of NH$_2$-glu-lys-glu-asn. Carboxypeptidase a digestion of CNBr peptide 2 showed a carboxyl terminal sequence of -tyr-ile-met-COOH. Protease digestion of BHA$_1$ followed by fractionation of the digest on Chromobeads P in pyridine acetate buffers results in the isolation of the chymotryptic overlap peptide NH$_2$-ile-met-glu-lys-COOH. This data shows that the sequence -ile-met-glu-lys- is only partially cleaved by cyanogen bromide. A similar sequence has been shown to be incompletely cleaved in the flagellin protein from *Bacillus subtilis* (Chang *et al.*,

Table 2

Amino Acid Composition of Cyanogen Bromide Fragments of BHA$_1$

	2	3	4	5	6	7	8	Total
Aspartic acid	15	4	7	3.9	3.1	3.4	1	37.4
Threonine	8.1	7.3	4	5.9	1.9	1.9	1	30.1
Serine	7	1.9	5.5	2.8	2.8	3.8	1	24.8
Glutamic acid	12.3	8.5	6.5	6.1	3.2	2.7	1	40.3
Proline	6.2	4.7	4	2.6	1	1		19.5
Glycine	10	4.1	5.3	5.4	3	3.9		31.7
Alanine	4.5	2	2	1	1	1		11.5
Valine	5.6	3.5	2.8	4	1.6			17.5
Methionine†	1		1	1	1	1	1	6
Isoleucine	9	3	1	2.6	3	3.2		21.8
Leucine	13.5	7	5	2.8	1.2	1.2	1	31.7
Tyrosine	3	1	1.9	1.7	2.1	1.2		10.9
Phenylalanine	*	1	3.8			1.8	1	7.6
Histidine	3.6	2	2.8	1.5				9.9
Lysine	7.2	4	5.6	2	2	1.8		22.6
Arginine	3	1	4	3.6		1		12.6
Cysteine‡	5.1	2.7	1.8					9.6
Total amino acids	114	58	64	47	27	29	9	346

†   as homoserine
*   analyses obscured by carbohydrate
‡   as S-carboxamidomethyl cysteine

Table 3

Amino Terminal Sequences of Cyanogen Fragments of BHA$_1$

CNBr Fragment

1	ASP – THR – ILE – CYS – ILE – GLY – – – – – –
2	ASP – THR – ILE – CYS – ILE – GLY – – – – – –
3	LYS – THR – GLU – GLY – THR – LEU – – – – –
4	GLU – LYS – GLU – ASN – PRO – ARG – – – – – –
5	LEU – ILE – ILE – TRYP – GLY – VAL – – – – – –
6	VAL – TRYP – LEU – THR – LYS – GLU – – – – – –
7	TRYP – ASP – THR – ILE – ASN – PHE – – – – – –
8	GLN – PHE – SER – TRYP – THR – LEU – – – – –

1976). Peptide 3 is the only cyanogen bromide peptide which lacks homoserine which suggests that it is derived from the carboxyl terminus of BHA_1. Peptide 2 which has the same amino terminal sequence as that of the undigested protein must represent the amino terminal 115 residues of BHA_1. Thus the following assignments may be made for the order of cyanogen bromide peptides in BHA_1:-

$$NH_2 - 2 - 4\ (5,6,7,8)\ 3 - COOH$$

Isolation of Methionine Overlap Peptides

Overlap peptides were isolated from a tryptic digest of whole BHA_1 which had been fully reduced and alkylated with ^{14}C-iodoacetamide. BHA_1 (100 nm) was digested with 2% TPCK trypsin (Worthington) (w/w) for 12 hr in 1% ammonium bicarbonate, digestion was terminated by addition of a 50 fold excess of phenylmethylsulphonylfluoride per mole of trypsin and the digest lyophilized. The digest was dissolved in 0.25 M acetic acid and insoluble material separated by centrifugation. Acid soluble peptides were fractionated on Sephadex G50 in 0.25 M acetic acid as shown in Figure 3. Fraction B from the G50 column was refractioned on QAE-Sephadex in pyridine acetate buffers and a methionine containing glycopeptide was isolated (Figure 4). Fraction D was subfractionated on the cation exchange resin Chromobeads P using pyridine acetate buffers

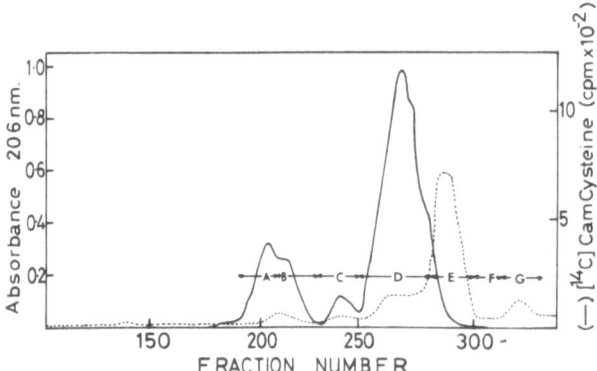

Figure 3

Fractionation of Tryptic Peptides of BHA_1

Peptides were separated on a 300 x 2 cm column of Sephadex G50 in 0.25 M acetic acid. The column effluent was monitored at 206 nm with a UVICORD III and aliquots were taken for measurement of radioactivity in $[^{14}C]$ carboxamidomethyl cysteine. Pools A-G were made as indicated and pools B and D were subfractionated as shown.

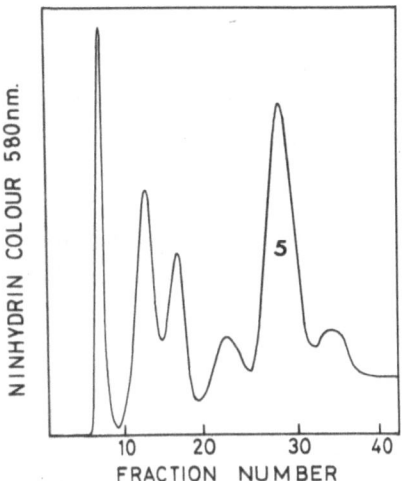

Figure 4

Fractionation of Large Tryptic Peptides of BHA$_1$

Peptides from pool B (Figure 3) were applied to a 0.9 x 15 cm column of QAE-Sephadex C-25 in 3% pyridine and the column was developed with the buffer system of Bradshaw *et al.* (1969). A portion of the effluent was monitored for ninhydrin positive material by the method of Herman and Vanaman (1975). The methionine containing peptide 5 located by amino acid analysis of pooled fractions.

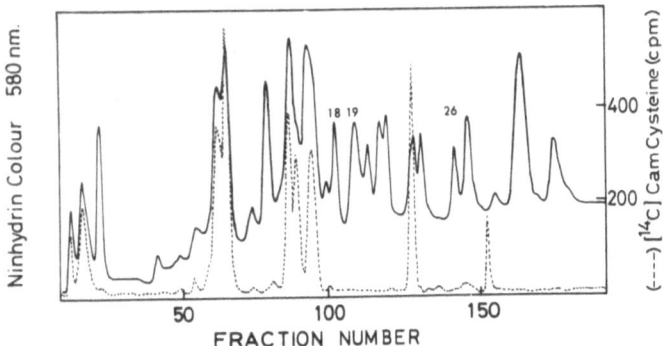

Figure 5

Fractionation of the Intermediate Size Tryptic Peptides of BHA

Peptides from pool D (Figure 3) were applied to a 0.9 x 30 cm column of Chromobeads P and the column was developed with a linear gradient of pyridine acetate buffers from 0.05 M, pH 2.4 to 2.0 M, pH 5 as described in the methods section. A portion of the column effluent was monitored for ninhydrin positive material by the method of Herman and Vanaman (1975) and radioactivity in [^{14}C] carboxamidomethyl cysteine was measured on aliquots of the fractions. Methionine containing peptides 18, 19 and 26 are indicated.

and an aliquot of the effluent was monitored for ninhydrin positive material (Klenk *et al.*, 1975) (Figure 5). Methionine containing peptides were identified by amino acid analysis of pooled fractions and these pools were subfractionated by column chromatography on the anion-exchange resin DA-X2 using pyridine acetate buffers or the peptides were fractionated by paper electrophoresis at pH 3.5 or 6.5 (Katz *et al.*, 1959). The acid insoluble tryptic peptides were fractionated on G50 Sephadex in 1% ammonium bicarbonate containing 10% propan-1-ol and a methionine peptide was located by amino acid analysis of pooled fractions (Figure 6). The amino acid composition of these peptides are shown in Table 4.

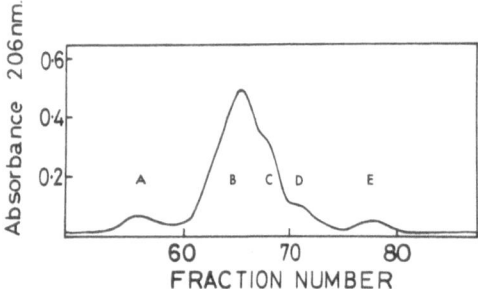

Figure 6

Fractionation of the Acid-Insoluble Tryptic Peptides of BHA$_1$

Peptides insoluble in 0.05 M pyridine acetate pH 2.4 were lyophilized and applied to a 300 x 2 cm column of Sephadex G50 in 0.2 M ammonia containing 10% propan-1-ol. The effluent was monitored at 206 nm with a UVICORD III. Peptide B contained methionine.

The determination of the carboxyl terminal amino acid sequence of the cyanogen bromide fragments was carried out on homoserine containing tryptic peptides isolated from protease digests of the fragments or by carboxypeptidase digestion of the whole cyanogen bromide fragment. The fractionation of these digests will be described separately. Results of sequence analysis of the overlap peptides are shown in Figure 7.

The alignment of cyanogen bromide peptides is summarized in Figure 7.

Discussion

A preliminary study of the structure of the hemagglutinin of influenza virus (Skehel and Waterfield, 1975) established the overall features of the glycopro-

Table 4

Amino Acid Composition of Methionine Containing Tryptic Peptides from BHA$_1$

	G50, B; QAE 5	Tr 18	Tr 19	Tr 26	â insol. G50 B
Aspartic acid	3			1	4
Threonine	2			1	3
Serine	2	2			2
Glutamic acid	5		1		3
Proline	1				1
Glycine	3	2			2
Alanine					1
Valine	1			1	
Methionine	1	1	1	1	2
Isoleucine	3	1	1		2
Leucine	1			1	3
Tyrosine	1				1
Phenylalynine					2
Histidine	2				
Lysine		1	1	1	1
Arginine	1				
Carbohydrate	+				

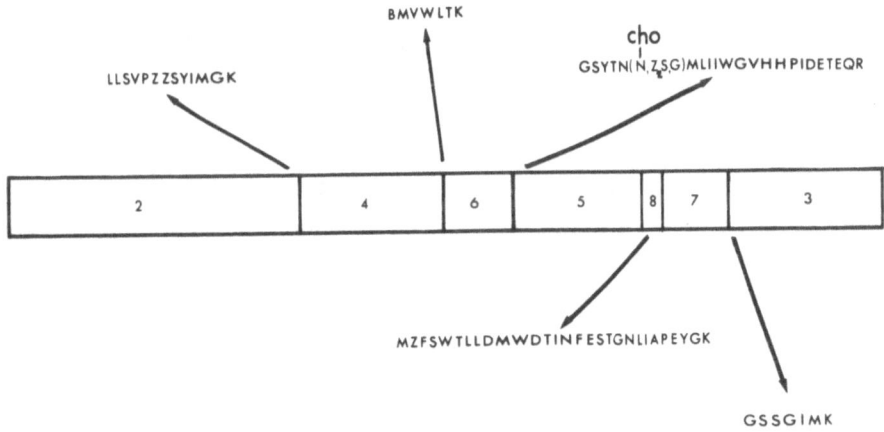

Figure 7

Alignment of Cyanogen Bromide Fragments of BHA$_1$

The sequence of overlap peptides and their location in the polypeptides are shown.

A	Ala	F	Phe	K	Lys	P	Pro	T	Thr
C	Cys	G	Gly	L	Leu	Q	Gln	V	Val
D	Asp	H	His	M	Met	R	Arg	Y	Tyr
E	Glu	I	Ile	N	Asn	S	Ser	Z	Glu or Gln

tein from the Bel 42 (H2N1) strain of virus. The present paper, together with the paper of McCauley *et al.* (1977, this volume) forms the next step in the elucidation of the primary structure of the HA from an Asian virus recombinant. This strain was selected for total sequence analysis based on a preliminary study of methionine content and cyanogen bromide cleavage pattern of the hemagglutinins from several strains. This work revealed that the Asian strains contained both the highest number of moles of methionine per mole of protein and had the most readily separable set of cyanogen bromide cleavage products. The amino acid composition of HA_1 obtained from virus disrupted with SDS was identical to that of BHA_1 obtained from Bromelain treated virus, The fractionation of the cyanogen bromide cleavage products of BHA_1 (Figures 1 and 2) showed that 8 distinct peptides were formed. Peptide 1 proved to be a partial cleavage product of peptides 2 and 4 showing that BHA_1 contained 7 unique peptides. The total amino acid composition of these 7 peptides matches the composition of the whole BHA_1 chain based on an amino acid content of 338 residues (excluding tryptophan). The separation of the cyanogen bromide fragments by gel exclusion chromatography was facilitated by the presence of carbohydrate side chains on peptides 2, 3 and 6. Peptide 3 contains 58 amino acids, is glycosylated and elutes from G100 before the 64 residue peptide 4 which is non-glycosylated. Similarily the glycosylated peptide 6 of 27 amino acids elutes prior to the non-glycosylated peptide 7 of 29 amino acid residues.

The alignment of the cyanogen bromide fragments is based on sequence analysis of overlapping methionine containing peptides and the carboxyl terminal sequence analysis of the cyanogen bromide fragments. Two large tryptic peptides (G50B, QAE 5 and acid insoluble peptide G50 B) have not been completely sequenced and the data available is only sufficient to assign probable positions for peptides 4, 5, 6, 7 and 8. The carboxyl terminal sequence of peptide 4 is still tentative (NH_2-arg asn met - COOH) and the overlap to peptide 8 is thus not conclusive.

These studies show that the BHA_1 chain contains 338 amino acids. Carbohydrate analysis gives a sugar composition of 24.4% which gives a total molecular weight of 50,000. The relative amounts of the sugars fucose, mannose, galactose and N-acetylglucosamine are similar to those of a serum glycoprotein. These sugars are all attached at asparagine residues and at least three separate sites of attachment are revealed by the cyanogen bromide fractionation. One attachment site is adjacent to the amino terminus and another is close to the carboxyl terminus.

Peptides 2, 3 and 4 contain 5, 3 and 2 cysteines respectively.These results make it possible to determine the complete amino acid sequence of the larger BHA_1 polypeptide chain. Similar studies of the smaller BHA_2 chain are described by McCauley *et al.* (1977, this volume)and together these results lay the ground work for a total sequence of the HA of one strain of influenza virus.

REFERENCES

BRADSHAW, R. A., GARNER, W. H. and GURD, F. R. N. (1969) J. Biol. Chem. *244*, 2149-2158.

BRAUER, A. W.. MARGOLIES, M. N. and HABER, E. (1975) Biochemistry *14*, 3029-3035.

CHANG, J. Y., DELANGE, R. J., SHAPER, J. H. and GLAZER, A. N. (1976) J. Biol. Chem. *251*, 695-700.

GROSS, E. and WITKOP, B. (1961) J. Am. Chem. Soc. *83*, 1510-1511.

HARTLEY, B. S. (1970) Biochem. J. *119*, 805-822.

HAY, A. J. (1974) Virology *60*, 398-418.

HERMAN, A. C. and VANAMAN, T. C. (1975) Anal. Biochem. *64*, 550-555.

KATZ, A. M., DREYER, W. J. and ANFINSEN, C. B. (1959) J. Biol. Chem. *234*, 2897-2900.

KLENK, H-D., ROTT, R., ORLICH, M. and BLÖDORN, J. (1975) Virology *68*, 426-439.

KLENK, H-D., SCHOLTISSEK, C. and ROTT, R. (1972) Virology *49*, 723-734.

LAINE, R. A., ESSELMAN, W. J. and SWEELEY, C. C. (1972) in 'Methods in Enzymology', XXVIII, 159-167.

LAVER, W. G. (1971) Virology *45*, 275-288.

LAVER, W. G. (1973) Advan. Virus Res. *18*, 57-103.

LAZAROWITZ, S. G., COMPANS, R. W. and CHOPPIN, P. W. (1971) Virology *46*, 828-843.

McCAULEY, J., SKEHEL, J. J. and WATERFIELD, M. D. (1977) this volume.

PISANO, J. J. and BRONZERT, T. J. (1969) J. Biol. Chem. *244*, 5597-5607.

SCHULZE, I. T. (1973) Advan. Virus Res. *18*, 1-55.

SKEHEL, J. J. and SCHILD, G. C. (1971) Virology *44*, 396-408.

SKEHEL, J. J. and WATERFIELD, M. D. (1975) Proc. Nat. Acad. Sci. USA. *72*, 93-97.

SMITHIES, O., GIBSON, D., FANNING, E. M., GOODFLEISH, R. M., GILMAN, J. G. and BALLANTYNE, D. L. (1971) Biochemistry *10*, 4912-4921.

SMYTH, D. G., STEIN, W. H. and MOORE, S. (1963) J. Biol. Chem. *238*, 227-234.

WILEY, D. C., SKEHEL, J. J. and WATERFIELD, M. D. (1977) Virology in press.

THE STRUCTURE OF THE SMALL POLYPEPTIDE CHAIN OF THE HEMAGGLUTININ OF AN ASIAN INFLUENZA VIRUS JAPAN 305/57 - BELLAMY/42 (H2N1)

J. McCauley, J. J. Skehel, and M. D. Waterfield

Summary

The hemagglutinin of the influenza virus variant A/Japan/305/57 - A/Bellamy/42 (H2N1) was isolated from virus particles following digestion with Bromelain (EC 3.4.22.4) and purified by sucrose density gradient centrifugation. The 2 component polypeptide chains BHA_1 and BHA_2 were separated, following full reduction and alkylation of cysteine residues by molecular sieving on Sephadex G-100. The smaller polypeptide chain BHA_2 was shown to contain 165 amino acid residues including 3 cysteine, 5 methionine, 6 arginine and 12 lysine residues. Six cyanogen bromide (CNBr) peptides which account for the total composition of the polypeptide have been purified by molecular sieving and ion exchange chromatography. These peptides have been aligned by sequence analysis of the CNBr peptides and by structural analysis of methionine containing protease generated overlap peptides. The amino terminal 9 residues of BHA_2 are shown to be hydrophobic. Residues 14-26 contain 2 tryptophan and 3 tyrosine residues. Glycine residues are located at positions 1, 4, 8, 12, 13, 16, 20, 23, 31 and 33. The 3 cysteine residues are located near the carboxyl terminus of the polypeptide.

The significance of these observations in understanding the structure of the hemagglutinin is discussed.

Introduction

The hemagglutinin (HA) spike of influenza virus is thought to be a trimer made up of 3 identical subunits having an apparent molecular weight of 75,000 on SDS polyacrylamide gels (Wiley et al., 1977; Skehel and Waterfield, 1975; Waterfield et al., 1977).

Each subunit is synthesized as a single polypeptide chain which is cleaved to form two disulfide linked polypeptide chains HA_1 and HA_2 having apparent molecular weights of 50,000 and 25,000 (Waterfield et al., 1977). The HA spike may be removed from the virus particles by the enzyme Bromelain (EC 3.4.22.4) liberating a polypeptide which has lost approximately 50-90 amino acids from the carboxyl terminus of HA_2, (Skehel and Waterfield, 1975). The bromelain released hemagglutinin (BHA) is composed of 2 disulfide linked chains BHA_1 and BHA_2 of apparent molecular weights 50,000 and 19,000.

This communication describes structural studies of the small polypeptide chain BHA_2 and forms part of a project to determine the primary amino acid sequence of the hemagglutinin. Similar structural studies on the larger polypeptide chain BHA_1 are described in the accompanying paper (Waterfield *et al.*, 1977).

Materials and Methods

Techniques for virus growth, protein purification and sequence analysis are described in Waterfield *et al.* (1977, this volume).

Tryptic Digestion

Tryptic digestion was carried out at $37^{\circ}C$ for 4 hours using an enzyme to substrate ratio of $1:100$ (w/w) at pH 8.5 in a pH stat.

Peptide Purification

Peptides were purified by cation exchange column chromatography on Chromobeads P (Technicon) using pyridine acetate buffers as described by Hewick *et al.* (1975). In some cases pyridine formate buffers (.04 M adjusted to pH 2 with formic acid as starting buffer and 3 M pyridine adjusted to pH 6 with formic acid as limiting buffer) were used to develop columns. The anion exchange resin DA-X2 (Durrum, Sunnyvale,Cal., USA.) was also used, employing the gradient system of Bornstein (1970).

Column effluents were monitored for radioactivity by scintillation counting of aliquots and for ninhydrin positive material by the method of Herman and Vanaman (1975). Pyridine was refluxed over ninhydrin and redistilled three times before use.

Solid Phase Sequence Analysis

Solid phase sequence analysis was carried out using an LKB 4020 sequencer with the methodology of Laursen *et al.* (1976).

Succinylation

Succinylation was performed by the method of Klotz (1967)

Cyanogen Bromide Cleavage

Cyanogen bromide cleavage was performed as described by Gross (1967) in 70% formic acid. Peptides were purified on Sephadex G75 Superfine followed by anion exchange chromatography as described in the text.

Results

Bromelain treatment of the influenza virus A/Bel 42 (H0N1) has been shown to release the hemagglutinin spike from the virus by a proteolytic cleavage at the carboxyl terminal region of the small polypeptide chain HA_2 resulting in the removal of approximately 50-90 amino acids, some of which are presumably associated with the lipid envelope (Skehel and Waterfield, 1975). Bromelain also removes the HA spike from the variant virus Jap/305 and the structural studies described here have been made on the shorter HA_2 polypeptide (BHA_2) which has been isolated from the cleaved HA molecule (BHA).

Table 1

Amino Acid Composition of BHA_2 from Japan/305/57

ASP	25.1
THR	6.3
SER	6.7
GLU	22.4
PRO	1.7
GLY	16.1
ALA	7.2
CYS	2.7
VAL	9.3
MET	4.3
ILE	4.1
LEU	12.2
TYR	8.7
PHE	8.8
HIS	3.9
LYS	12.4
ARG	5.9

Total 159 residues

Molecular Weight and Amino Acid Composition

The molecular weight of BHA_2 has been derived from gel filtration in guanidine hydrochloride and from structural studies described later. BHA_2 contains approximately 9% carbohydrate and is eluted from columns of Sepharose 4B in 6 M guanidine hydrochloride pH 4 as if it were a polypeptide of molecular weight 19,200 (McCauley, Skehel and Waterfield, 1977, unpublished observations). This data is compatible with a polypeptide chain of approximately 160 amino acids. The amino acid analysis of BHA_2 shown in Table 1 is based on this figure, which would indicate that the polypeptide should contain 2.7 (3) cysteine, 4.7 (5) methionine, 6 arginine and 12 lysine residues.

Cyanogen Bromide Cleavage of BHA_2

BHA_2 was treated with cyanogen bromide in 70% formic acid for 18 hr, the digest was lyophilized and taken up in ammonium hydroxide containing 10% propanol and fractionated on Sephadex G-75 superfine. The elution profile is shown in Figure 1. Three pools were made (2, 3 + 4 and 5 + 6) and each was separately fractionated on the anion exchange resin DA x 2 using pyridine acetate buffers. Four cyanogen bromide peptides were purified using the combination of Sephadex G75 and DA x 2 ion exchange columns (peptides 2, 4, 5 and 6). One cyanogen bromide peptide which was insoluble in ammonia propanol (peptide 1) and another soluble peptide (6) could not be obtained completely pure by these techniques.

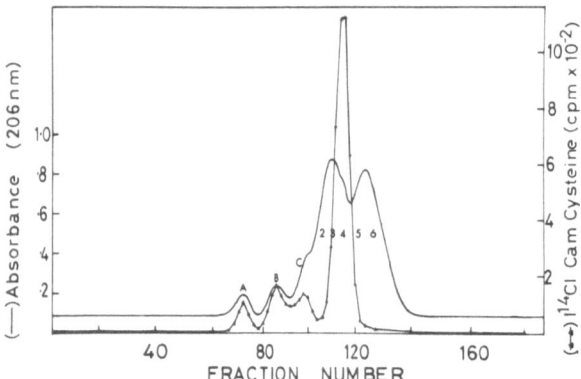

Figure 1

Fractionation of cyanogen bromide digest of BHA_2 on Sephadex G-75 superfine (2 meters x 1.5 cm) in 0.01 M ammonium hydroxide containing 10% propan-1-ol. Absorbence at 206 nm was monitored with a UVICORD III and radioactivity in aliquots of each fraction was measured by scintillation counting.

Structural Analysis of Cyanogen Bromide Peptides

The amino acid compositions of 5 of the cyanogen bromide peptides are given in Table 2. Amino acid sequence analysis of intact BHA_2 in the automatic sequencer revealed a methionine residue at position 17 and the composition of peptide 1 is derived from this sequence analysis since this peptide is extremely hydrophobic, having only 2 charged residues, and has not been obtained pure. Peptide 4 contains all the cysteine residues and a blocked amino terminus. Peptide 2 contains 4 of the 8 tyrosine residues of the polypeptide. Peptides 5 and 6 are the most basic having 4 and 5 lysine plus arginine residues respectively. Peptide 3 has proved extremely difficult to purify. This peptide is the only one which lacks homoserine and contains proline. The amino terminal sequence of peptides 2, 4, 5 and 6 was determined by liquid or solid phase sequence analysis and are the amino terminal regions shown in Figure 2. The amino term-

CB1 GLY–LEU–PHE–GLY–ALA–ILE–ALA–GLY–PHE–ILE–GLU–GLY–GLY–TRP–GLU–GLY–MET

CB2 VAL–ASP–GLY–TRP–TYR–GLY–TYR–

CB3 ASN–SER–VAL–LYS

CB4 GLN–LEU–ARG–ASX–ASX–VAL–LYS–GLX–LEU

CB5 GLU–ASX–GLX–ARG–THR–LEU–ASX–PHE–HIS–

CB6 ASN–THR–GLN–PHE–GLN–ALA–VAL–GLY–LYS–

Figure 2

Amino terminal sequences of cyanogen bromide peptides of BHA$_2$.

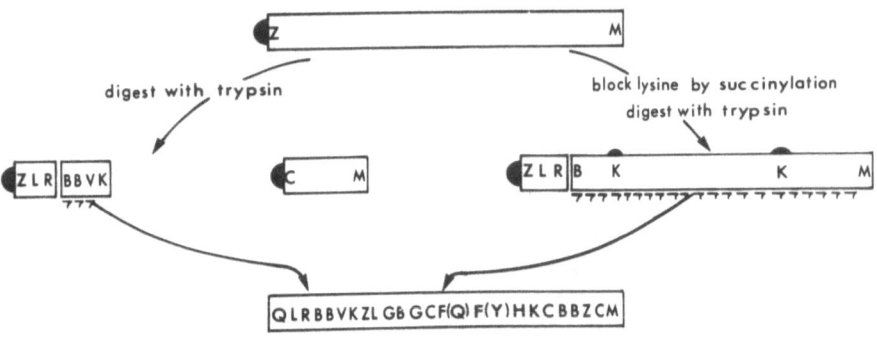

Figure 3

Outline of the determination of the amino acid sequence of cyanogen bromide peptide 4. Details are given in the text.

A	Ala	F	Phe	K	Lys	P	Pro	T	Thr
C	Cys	G	Gly	L	Leu	Q	Gln	V	Val
D	Asp	H	His	M	Met	R	Arg	Y	Tyr
E	Glu	I	Ile	N	Asn	S	Ser	Z	Glu or Gln

inal sequence of peptide 4 was determined by a different strategy (outlined in Figure 3) since the amino terminus was blocked to Edman degradation when isolated by the techniques described above. Tryptic digestion of peptide 4 followed by fractionation on ion exchange columns resulted in recovery of 3 peptides, however two of these peptides had blocked amino termini. One blocked peptide contained homoserine and must be derived from the carboxyl terminus of 4. The second blocked peptide contained one glutamic acid, one leucine and one arginine residue. Since the original peptide 4 contained only one arginine residue, the lysine side chains were blocked by succinylation and the modified peptide was then coupled through the carboxyl terminal homoserine to aminopropyl glass and subjected to solid phase sequence analysis. The results are summarized in Figure 3. The amino terminal sequence has been tentatively deduced as glutamine-leucine-arginine on the basis that the peptide has become blocked due to cyclization of glutamine to pyrrolidine-carboxylic acid. The arginine is placed at the carboxyl terminus since the tri-peptide (glx, leu, arg) was obtained by tryptic cleavage. Cyclization of an amino terminal S-carboxyamidomethyl cysteine residue generated by tryptic cleavage probably explains the failure in sequence analysis of the carboxyterminal tryptic peptide. These results illustrate the problems of cyclization of amino terminal glutamine and S-carboxyamido-methyl cysteine which could have been exaggerated by the techniques of column chromatography used to purify peptides.

The carboxyl terminal cyanogen bromide peptide (3) has proved difficult to purify and only the four amino terminal residues have been sequenced by analysis of a mixture of peptides 2 and 3.

The amino acid compositions of the cyanogen bromide peptides are shown in Table 2.

Isolation and Structural Characterization of Tryptic Peptides of BHA$_2$

Tryptic peptides have been isolated from a digest of BHA$_2$ in order to purify methionine containing overlap peptides and to confirm the amino acid sequence determined by analysis of cyanogen bromide peptides. BHA$_2$ was digested with TPCK trypsin for 4 hours and the digest fractionated on Chromobeads P cation exchange resin with a gradient of increasing ion strength and pH using pyridine acetate buffers. The effluent from the column was continuously monitored for ninhydrin positive material and the results are shown in Figure 4. An aliquot of each peak was analyzed by paper electrophoresis and peaks containing more than one peptide were refractionated. Acidic peptides were chromatographed on the anion exchange resin DA x 2 using pyridine acetate gradients and basic peptides were rechromatographed on Chromobeads P using pyridine formate gradients. These methods resulted in the purification of nineteen peptides.

187

Table 2

Amino Acid Compositions of Cyanogen Bromide Peptides

	CNBr1†	CNBr2	CNBr3	CNBr4	CNBr5	CNBr6	Total
CYS*	(0)	0.0	0.0	2.8 (3)	0.0 (0)	0.0 (0)	2.8
ASP	(0)	7.9	2.6	4.7 (5)	6.2 (6)	3.9 (4)	25.3
THR	(0)	2.1	1.0	0.2 (0)	1.0 (1)	1.0 (1)	5.3
SER	(0)	3.9	1.9	0.7 (0)	1.0 (1)	1.4 (1)	8.9
GLU	(2)	4.5	3.2	4.2 (4)	2.7 (3)	5.4 (5)	22.0
PRO	(0)	0.3	2.3	0.2 (0)	0.0 (0)	0.0 (0)	2.8
GLY	(6)	5.6	3.4	2.4 (2)	0.3 (0)	1.6 (1)	19.3
ALA	(2)	3.1	1.3	0.2 (0)	0.0 (0)	1.2 (1)	7.8
VAL	(0)	4.2	1.5	0.9 (1)	2.2 (2)	0.8 (1)	9.6
MET‡	(1)	1.0	0.3	1.0 (1)	1.0 (1)	1.0 (1)	5.3
ILE	(2)	2.2	1.0	0.0 (0)	0.0 (0)	0.3 (0)	5.5
LEU	(1)	0.7	1.8	2.0 (2)	2.2 (2)	3.0 (3)	10.7
TYR	(0)	4.3	1.4	1.2 (1)	0.7 (1)	0.0 (0)	7.6
PHE	(2)	1.5	0.8	2.1 (2)	1.4 (1)	2.4 (2)	10.2
HIS	(0)	1.9	0.3	0.9 (1)	1.1 (1)	0.0 (0)	4.2
LYS	(0)	4.1	1.2	1.8 (2)	2.1 (2)	2.5 (3)	11.8
ARG	(0)	0.2	0.7	1.1 (1)	2.1 (2)	2.0 (2)	6.1
TRP☆	(1)	(?1)	N.D.	N.D. (0)	N.D. (0)	N.D. (0)	
Total	(17)	49	25	25.3 (25)	23 (23)	26.5 (25)	165.2

*   Cysteine determined as s-carboxymethylcysteine.   ☆   Tryptophan not determined

‡   Methionine determined as homoserine   †   CNBr1 not isolated

The figures in parentheses are the numbers of each amino acid found in the sequence.

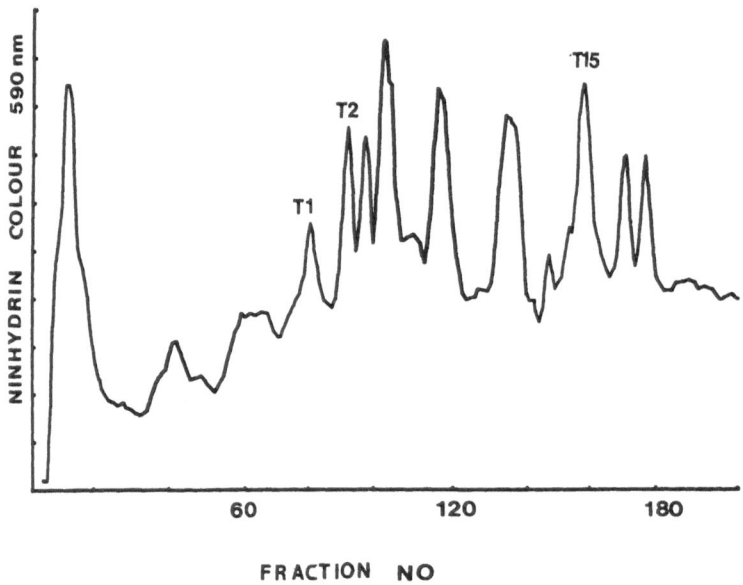

Figure 4

Purification of tryptic peptides of BHA₂ by chromatography on a cation exchange column in pyridine acetate buffers. Absorbence at 590 nm was monitored by the method of Herman and Vanaman (1975), other details are given in the methods section. Methionine containing peptides T1, T2 and T15 are indicated.

Three methionine containing peptides were purified (T1, T2 and T15) of which 2 had blocked amino termini. The amino acid composition of the peptides T1 and T2 and the amino acid sequence of T15 which was determined by the dansyl Edman technique are shown in Table 3. The sequence of the other tryptic peptides has been determined by the dansyl Edman technique or by solid phase sequence analysis.

Table 3

Amino Acid Composition and Partial Sequences of Methionine Overlap Peptides of BHA₂ from Japan/305/57

T2 GLN(GLX₂,MET,ASX,GLY,THR,PHE,VAL,ALA,LYS)

T1 (CmCYS₂,ASX₃,GLX,MET,VAL,SER,LYS)

T15 MET − GLN − LEU − ARG

Alignment of Cyanogen Bromide Fragment of BHA$_2$

Amino acid sequence analysis of whole BHA$_2$ in the liquid phase sequencer has given the sequence of cyanogen bromide peptide 1 which covers residues 1 to 17 (Figure 2). The same analysis showed that cyanogen bromide peptide 2 could be placed next to peptide 1. Peptide 3 lacks homoserine and is presumably carboxyl terminal. Three methionine containing tryptic peptides have been isolated and preliminary structural data can be used to align the remaining cyanogen bromide fragments (3, 4, 5 and 6). The carboxyl terminal sequence of cyanogen bromide peptide 5 was (-arg-glx-met), and the amino terminal sequence of cyanogen bromide peptide 6 was (asn-thr-gln-phe-gln-ala-gly-lys). These two cyanogen bromide peptides can be aligned by the blocked tryptic overlap peptide T2 (see Table 3) which has a composition compatible with tryptic cleavage between the arginine and glutamic acid or glutamine residue at the carboxyl terminus of peptide 5 and tryptic cleavage following the lysine which is residue 8 in cyanogen bromide peptide 6. Presumably cyclization of an amino terminal glutamine has blocked tryptic peptide 2. Thus the cyanogen bromide peptides can be aligned NH$_2$-1-2-? -(6-5)-? -3-COOH. The location of peptide 4 can be assigned from the determination of the amino terminal sequence of peptide 3 which is asn-ser-val-lys, and knowledge of the carboxyl terminal sequence of peptide 4 which is cys-asx-asx-(glx-cys)met. These two sequences are compatible with an overlap peptide having the composition of tryptic peptide T1. This peptide is blocked, which is presumably due to cyclization of the amino terminal S-carboxyamidomethyl cysteine residue. These results suggest the alignment NH$_2$-1-2(6-5)-? -(4-3)-COOH.

The final alignment of the peptides can be tentatively made using the information that peptide 3 is carboxyl terminal and the sequence at the carboxyl terminus of cyanogen bromide peptide 6 is (lys-met) while the amino terminus of peptide 4 is (gln-leu-arg), these sequences together are compatible with the overlap peptide T15 which has the sequence met-gln-leu-arg. This assignment must be regarded as tentative until all complete sequence data is available but the data is compatible with a single arrangement of cyanogen bromide peptides of the order 1-2-6-5-4-3. The results are summarized in Figure 5.

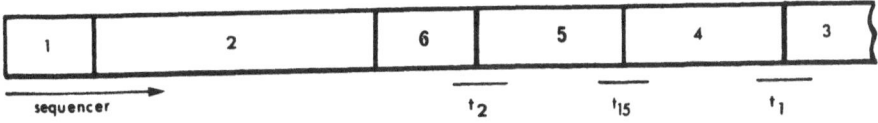

Figure 5

Alignment of cyanogen bromide peptides of BHA$_2$. Experimental details are given in the text. The location of tryptic peptides T1, T2 and T15 are shown.

Discussion

This study of the structure of the small glycopolypeptide of the influenza virus variant Jap/305/57 - Bel/42 (H2N1) forms part of a project to determine the total primary amino acid sequence of the hemagglutinin of this virus. In this paper results of the structural analysis of the glycopolypeptide BHA_2, which was purified from Bromelain released hemagglutinin, are described. This glyco- polypeptide BHA_2 differs from the native glycopolypeptide HA_2 by approxi- mately 50-90 amino acids which have been cleaved from the carboxyl-terminus during the Bromelain digestion. The precise determination of the molecular weight of BHA_2 can be made from the structural studies described here in com- bination with determinations of carbohydrate content and apparent Stokes radius which have previously been carried out (Waterfield *et al.*, unpublished results, 1977). The glycopolypeptide BHA_2 contains 9% carbohydrate and elutes from a Sepharose 4B column in 6 M guanidine hydrochloride as a poly- peptide of apparent molecular weight 19,200. This indicates that the molecular weight of the polypeptide portion of the chain is 17,500. This would be com- patible with a polypeptide of 159 amino acids of average molecular weight 128. Amino acid analysis of BHA_2 shown in Table 1 is calculated on 159 residues, having the average amino acid molecular weight of 128. The composition of BHA_2 based on 159 residues predicts that BHA_2 should have 2.7 cysteine, 4.7 methionine, 6 arginine and 12 lysine residues. The structural studies indi- cate that the chain can be cleaved by cyanogen bromide to give 6 peptides. The cyanogen bromide peptide CNBr 4 has been purified and shown to contain 3 cysteine residues. Tryptic digests of BHA_2 have been shown to contain nineteen soluble peptides including free lysine, free arginine and one peptide lacking lysine or arginine. These peptides have been recovered in variable yields and although the predicted number of peptides expected after tryptic cleavage is nineteen it is not possible to be certain that some peptides have not been found until sequence analysis is finished. However at this stage of analysis all the data is compatible with a polypeptide of 159 residues having carbohydrate attached giving a total molecular weight of 19,200.

Cyanogen bromide cleavage of BHA_2 has been performed and four pure pep- tides and one partially pure peptide have been purified by a combination of molecular sieving and ion exchange chromatography. The amino terminal pep- tide has not been recovered since it is hydrophobic and insoluble in most buf- fers. Separate experiments have shown that the peptide does not aggregate in 6 M urea containing 0.2 M formic acid since it is eluted in a position correspond- ing to its predicted molecular weight. However during removal of the urea the peptide becomes quite intractable.

The carboxyl terminal cyanogen bromide peptide has not yet been recovered pure but some sequence information has been obtained, from a partially pure preparation, by sequencer analysis of a mixture of CNBr-2 and CNBr-3. The cyanogen bromide peptides have been tentatively aligned using incomplete overlap data. Further structural analysis should inequivocally establish the order of these peptides.

The present study shows several interesting features of the BHA_2 polypeptide. The amino terminal region of 17 residues contains only 2 charged amino acids and is extremely hydrophobic. Cleavage of a polypeptide precursor of the hemagglutinin is necessary to form the 2 polypeptide chains HA_1 and HA_2 and is also essential for activation of viral infectivity. This cleavage has been shown to take place at the carboxyl terminus of HA_1 and to result in the generation of the amino terminus of HA_2 (Skehel and Waterfield, 1975). Thus the cleavage results in the generation of a hydrophobic amino terminus on HA_2. A comparison of hydrophobic regions from proteins of known sequence with the amino terminal 9 residues of BHA_2 by the method of Segrest et al. (1974) shows that this region is as hydrophobic as regions of other polypeptides known to be associated with lipid membranes. It has been shown by Gething et al. (1977) that the activation cleavage of the putative fusion factor 'F' of Sendai virus also leads to the generation of a new amino terminus with an analogous hydrophobic sequence to that found at the amino terminus of BHA_2. Thus in both influenza and Sendai virus the protease activation of infectivity (and fusion in the case of Sendai) is associated with the generation of an amino terminal hydrophobic region which was previously an internal sequence of the precursor polypeptide chain. It is possible that cleavage prior to insertion of the HA polypeptide in the membrane, which would generate a polypeptide with 2 hydrophobic regions (one at the NH_2-terminus of HA_2 and another at the COOH-terminus of HA_2) might interfere with the orientation of the spike in the membrane.

The structures of the newly generated hydrophobic regions suggest that they may be involved in interactions with host cell membranes during infection (see Gething et al., 1977, this volume), however no experimental evidence is yet available to support this concept. The hydrophobic region at the amino terminus of HA_2 is followed by a region containing several aromatic amino acids (see Figure 2). This region could be concerned in the optical changes associated with cleavage of the precursor HA. The 3 cysteine residues are located within 12 amino acids close to the carboxyl terminus of BHA_2. The spacing of 2 of these cysteines which have 3 residues between them is identical to the spacing of 2 cysteines in BHA_1 (Waterfield et al., unpublished results).

These studies form an intermediate stage in the determination of the amino acid sequence of the HA molecule. It is anticipated that a further understanding of the function of HA will result from such studies in conjunction with studies of the 3 dimensional structure and biology.

REFERENCES

BORNSTEIN, P. (1970) Biochemistry 9, 2408-2421.

GETHING, M-J., WHITE, J. M. and WATERFIELD, M. D. (1977) this volume.

GROSS, E. (1967) Methods in Enzymology 11, 238-255.

HERMAN, A. C. and VANAMAN, T. C. (1975) Anal. Biochem. 64, 550-555.

HEWICK, R. M., FRIED, M. and WATERFIELD, M. D. (1975) Virology 66, 408-419.

KLOTZ, I. M. (1967) Methods in Enzymology 11, 576-580.

LAURSEN, R. A., BONNER, A. G. and HORN, M. J. (1976) in 'Instrumentation in Amino Acid Sequence Analysis' (ed. Perham, R.) Acad. Press.

SEGREST, J. P. and FELDMAN, R. J. (1974) J. Mol. Biol. 87, 853-858.

SKEHEL, J. J. and WATERFIELD, M. D. (1975) Proc. Nat. Acad. Sci. USA. 72, 93-97.

WATERFIELD, M. D., SKEHEL, J. J., NAKASHIMA, Y., GURNETT, A. and BILHAM, T. (1977) this volume.

WILEY, D., SKEHEL, J. J. and WATERFIELD, M. D. (1977) Virology in press.

STUDIES ON THE PRIMARY STRUCTURE OF THE HEMAGGLUTININ FROM AN H3N2 VARIANT A/MEMPHIS/102/72

Theo A. A. Dopheide and Colin W. Ward

Introduction

Pathogens responsible for chronic or repeated infections evade the immune response by either the adsorption of host antigens, as in schistosomiasis (Clegg,
1974), the release of soluble surface antigens, as with maleria, *Babesia* and
nematode infections, (Wilson, 1974) or by a process of antigenic variation, as
in trypanosomiasis and influenza. In trypanosomiasis, antigenic variation is
phenotypic and involves the sequential expression of alternative genes (Bridgen
and Cross, 1976). In influenza, antigenic variation was also once thought to be
phenotypic, the virion supposedly possessing a mosaic of antigens variably
exposed in different strains (see Fazekas de St. Groth, 1970; Webster and Laver,
1975, for reviews). However the wealth of information published on the biology,
structure, chemistry and immunology of influenza virus over the last fifteen
years has established beyond doubt that antigenic variability in influenza is
genetic (Kilbourne, 1975).

The nature of this antigenic variation (major shifts to new sub-types every ten
to fifteen years and minor drifts within each sub-type every two or three years),
the confinement of this variation to the two surface glycoproteins (neuraminidase and hemagglutinin) which change independently, and the evidence implic-
ating the hemagglutinin as the more important of these two antigens, have been
extensively reviewed (Skehel, 1974; Webster and Laver, 1975; Schild and
Dowdle, 1975).

There is less general agreement about the mechanism behind this antigenic variation. Antigenic drift is thought to result from the selection of antigenically new
mutants during the transmission of viruses through partially immune populations. Peptide maps show small differences in the hemagglutinins of such viruses
(Webster and Laver, 1975). Whether this drift occurs in a random manner or in-

volves the sequential replacement of hydrophobic amino acids of increasing side chain surface area (Fazekas de St. Groth, 1970, 1975) remains to be established. There is even greater dispute regarding the mechanism of antigenic shift and the origin of new pandemics. Fazekas de St. Groth (1970, 1975) has proposed that new pandemics arise by mutation from pre-existing human influenza viruses via so-called bridging strains, while Webster and Laver (1975) suggest that new pandemics may arise by genetic recombination between human and animal influenza viruses.

Comparative amino acid sequences of hemagglutinins from animal viruses and human sub-types are required to characterize the nature of the hemagglutinin antigenic determinants (Virelizier *et al.*, 1974; Laver *et al.*, 1974) and to resolve the dispute over the mechanism of antigenic variation.

This laboratory is currently investigating the structure of the hemagglutinin from the Hong Kong variant A/Memphis/102/72 (H3N2). In this report some of our recent findings on the molecular weight, carbohydrate composition, amino acid composition and amino acid sequence are presented and compared with the published data for other influenza strains.

Materials and Methods

The virus strain used, the procedures employed in virus cultivation and purification, hemagglutinin isolation and separation into heavy (HA_1) and light (HA_2) chains, acrylamide gel electrophoresis and amino acid and carbohydrate analyses have been described (Ward and Dopheide, 1976).

Amino acid sequences were determined by the Peterson-modified Edman procedure (Peterson *et al.*, 1972). Amino acids were generallly identified as the Dansyl-derivatives (Hartley, 1970) but PTH-derivatives were also identified as described by Inglis and Nicholls (1973) for acid/amide assignments.

Results and Discussion

Molecular Weight

The reported molecular weight of the hemagglutinin polypeptides show wide variation (Table 1) which may reflect differences in the amino acid composition of the original HA, differences in the position of cleavage (Schulze, 1970), differences in the amount of carbohydrate attached to the polypeptide chains (Compans *et al.*, 1970) or differences in the methods used to determine these molecular weights (Ward and Dopheide, 1976).

Table 1

Apparent Molecular Weights of Hemagglutinin Chains

Virus		HA_1	HA_2	Conditions
A/Bel (H0)		65,000	25,000	5% SDS gels
		65,000	23,000	5% SDS gels
		60,000	21,000	7.5% SDS gels
		58,000	28,000	7.5% SDS gels
	(a)	47,000	-	Gel filtration in 6 M GuHCl
A/WSN (H0)		50,000	25,000	8% SDS gels
		50,000	30,000	7.5% SDS gels
		49,000	30,000	7.5% SDS gels
A/Mem/102/72 (H3)	(b)	94,000	34,000	3% SDS gels
		73,000	32,600	4% SDS gels
		66,000	31,000	5% SDS gels
		56,000	30,000	7.5% SDS gels
		53,400	30,000	10% SDS gels
		52,000	30,000	12.5% SDS gels
		51,000	30,000	15% SDS gels
		47,000	-	Ultracentrifugation in 6.0 M GuHCl
A/FPV (Hav1)		49,000	32,000	10% SDS gels
		49,000	28,000	10% SDS gels
		46,000	29,000	10% SDS gels
B/Lee		63,000	27,000	5% SDS gels
	(c)	54,000	27,000	13% SDS gels

Table based on that from White (1974) with additional data from (a) Webster (1970) (b) Ward and Dopheide (1976) and (c) Tobita and Kilbourne (1975).

With two exceptions, all molecular weight estimations for HA_1 and HA_2 have been obtained by SDS gel electrophoresis, a procedure that consistantly leads to overestimations when applied to glycoproteins with more than 10% carbohydrate (Segrest and Jackson, 1972). The degree of overestimation decreases as the acrylamide gel concentration is increased and this is well illustrated by the data in Table 1. As the gel concentration increases, the apparent molecular weight approaches the true molecular weight which on ultracentrifugal analysis (Ward and Dopheide, 1976) or gel filtration (Webster, 1970) in 6 M guanidine HCl, was shown to be 47,000 for Mem/72 HA_1 and Bel/42 HA_1 respectively.

Although varying experimental conditions account for a great deal of the variation in reported molecular weights, other factors such as differences in carbohydrate content also contribute. When examined under identical conditions the hemagglutinin subunits of Bel/42 (HO) and Singapore/57 (H2) gave different apparent molecular weights (Skehel and Waterfield, 1975).

Carbohydrate Composition

The carbohydrate compositions of Mem/72 HA_1 and HA_2 are shown in Table 2. Both chains are glycosylated but most of the carbohydrate is on the heavy chain. For a molecular weight of 47,000 (Ward and Dopheide, 1976), the carbohydrate content of HA_1 totals 11,450 daltons and puts the apoprotein molecular weight at 35,500. Only four sugars were present in HA_1, N-acetylglucosamine, galactose, mannose and fucose with molar ratios 3.8/2/6.6/1. The only other reported carbohydrate analysis in the literature is for Bel/42 HA_1 which had a total carbohydrate content of 10,200 - 12,000 daltons and the same four sugars but in different molar ratios of 6.4/1.2/4.0/1 (Laver, 1971).

Table 2

Carbohydrate Composition of A/Mem/102/72 Hemagglutinin Chains

Sugar	Residues/Mole	
	HA_1	HA_2
N-Acetylglucosamine	19	7
Galactose	10	0.4
Mannose	33	0.6
Fucose	5	0.3

Mem/72 HA_1 contains about three times as much N-acetylglucosamine as HA_2, which is similar to the ratios of radiolabelled glucosamine found incorporated in Bel/42 hemagglutinin chains (Stanley and Haslam, 1971).

Mem/72 HA_2, molecular weight 29,700 (Ward and Dopheide, 1976), contains only N-acetylglucosamine for a carbohydrate content of 1400 daltons and an apoprotein molecular weight of 28,300. The presence of the other sugars in less than molar quantities may result from either slight contamination with some HA_1 (although ratios differed) or from heterogeneity in the carbohydrate groups of HA_2 (Gottschalk, 1969).

The presence of N-acetylglucosamine and the absence of N-acetylgalactosamine and xylose suggests the carbohydrate is all attached via N-glycosidic linkage to asparagine and none by O-glycosidic linkage to serine or threonine (Neuberger *et al.*, 1972). So far the amino acid sequence of one glycopeptide (CNBr 3) from HA_1 has been determined. It had a glycosylated asparagine residue in the sequence: Ile-Thr-Pro-*ASN*-Gly-Ser-Ile-Pro- and conformed to the general pattern Asn-X-$\frac{Ser}{Thr}$ found with other glycoproteins (Neuberger *et al.*, 1972). This glycopeptide also conformed to the pattern that if residue X, in the sequence Asn-X-Y, is not hydrophilic, then the sugar moiety is of the simple type containing only mannose and N-acetylglucosamine (Jackson and Hirs, 1970; Funatsu *et al.*, 1971). In CNBr 3 the X residue is Gly and the sugar unit had the composition Mannose$_5$. N-acetylglucosamine$_2$.

Amino Acid Composition

The amino acid compositions of Mem/72 hemagglutinin chains are shown in Table 3. Both chains contain four methionines and eight cysteines per mole of protein. The most striking difference between the two chains is the proline content; HA_2 has only 3 residues of proline compared to 21 in HA_1 and a similar proline ratio has been reported for the hemagglutinin chains of Bel/42 (Laver, 1971; Stanley *et al.*, 1973; Skehel and Waterfield, 1975).

For direct comparison, Table 3 also contains the amino acid composition of Bel/42 HA_1 and HA_2 taken from Skehel and Waterfield (1975) and recalculated using a molecular weight for Bel/42 HA_1 of 47,000 (Webster, 1970), with 11 to 12,000 daltons of carbohydrate (Laver, 1971) and an apoprotein molecular weight of 35-36,000 which corresponds to approximately 330 amino acid residues.

Amino Acid Sequences

Partial amino acid sequences for the N-terminal regions of HA_1 and HA_2 from different strains of influenza have recently been published (Skehel and Waterfield, 1975; Bucher *et al.*, 1976). In view of the many differences seen in the peptide maps of the hemagglutinin chains of different virus sub-types (Webster and Laver, 1975) the constancy of the HA_2 N-terminal sequences in all strains was surprising.

The HA_1 N-terminal sequences for H0 and H2 viruses were also very similar, a fact which supports Fazekas de St. Groth's (1970, 1975) contention that the A2 pandemic originated by mutation from A0 viruses. However they are obviously different from the H3 heavy chains. We have found that Mem/72 HA_1 has a blocked end group which may be a general feature of all the H3 heavy chains. Skehel and Waterfield (1975) published light chain N-terminal sequences

Table 3

Amino Acid Compositions of HA$_1$ and HA$_2$ from A/Bel/42 (HO) and A/Memphis/102/72 (H3)

Residue	HA$_1$		HA$_2$	
	Bel/42	Mem/72	Bel/42	Mem/72
Lys	18	15	18	16
His	8	6	5	6
Arg	14	14	6	11
Asp	38	44	35	32
Thr	23	29	12	13
Ser	28	30	21	13
Glu	35	25	31	33
Pro	18	21	5	3
Gly	25	29	23	23
Ala	16	14	13	15
½ Cys	7	8	5	8
Val	18	21	15	10
Met	2	4	6	4
Ile	21	22	15	21
Leu	26	22	21	19
Tyr	14	11	12	8
Phe	11	11	10	11
Trp	ND*	5	ND*	4

Composition expressed as residues per mole protein. Mem/72 data from Ward and Dopheide (1976), Bel/42 data recalculated from Skehel and Waterfield (1975).
*   ND = Not determined.

for five different virus strains, but heavy chain sequences for only three. No heavy chain data was presented for the two H3 viruses X-31 and MRC-11, possibly because their HA$_1$ N-terminal residues are also blocked.

If a blocked HA$_1$ N-terminus is a characteristic of the Hong Kong (H3) subtype then the HA$_1$ of the two putative progenitors of the Hong Kong pandemic, A/equine/Miami/1/63 and A/Duck/Ukraine/1/63 (Laver and Webster, 1973), should also have a blocked end group. This has recently been shown to be so (Laver and Webster, 1977 this volume). We have cleaved Mem/72 HA$_1$ at the methionine residues with cyanogen bromide and obtained five peptides. CN-1 had an apoprotein molecular weight of approximately 15,000 and contains most, but not all, of the carbohydrate from HA_1. It has a blocked end group and is probably the N-terminal peptide.

CN-2 has a molecular weight of about 12,000, the N-terminal sequence Pro-Asn-Asn-Asp-Asn-Phe-Asp-Lys- and the C-terminal sequence Val-Met. The sequence of this peptide is now almost completed and will be published elsewhere.

The sequence of CN-3 has been completely determined. It contains 52 amino acid residues, has the N-terminal sequence Arg-Ser-Asp-Ala-Pro-Ile-Gly-Thr-CmCys-Ile- and the C-terminal sequence Lys-Leu-Ala-Thr-Gly-Met. It contains a glycosylated asparagine residue as already discussed in the section on carbohydrate and three CmCys residues.

CN-4 and CN-5 are both octapeptides with the sequences Arg-Thr-Gly-Lys-Ser-Ser-Ile-Met and Arg-Asn-Val-Pro-Glu-Lys-Gln-Thr respectively. CN-5 is the C-terminal peptide. The presence of Thr as the C-terminal residue was unexpected in view of the proteolytic cleavage at this point in the production of HA_1 and HA_2 (Choppin and Compans, 1975). Nothing is known of the nature of the proteolytic enzymes operating in the allantoic sac of the chick embryo but

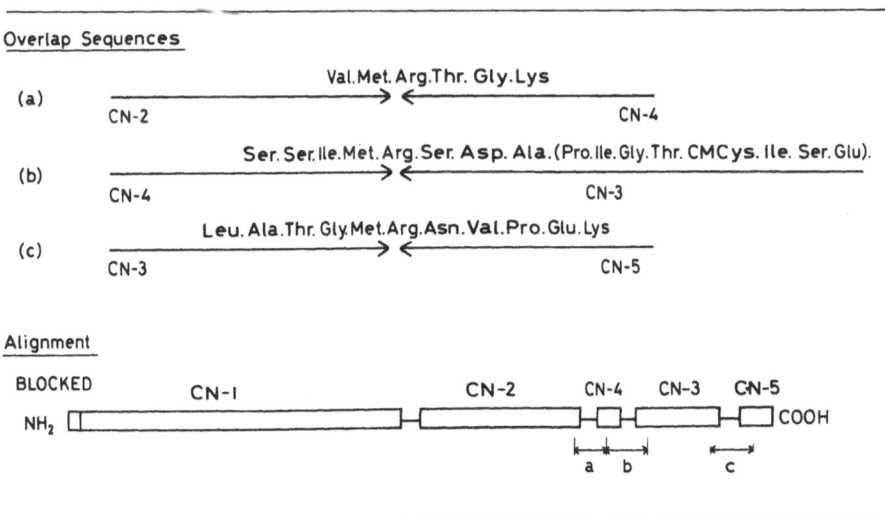

ALIGNMENT OF CNBr PEPTIDES

Figure 1

Methionine overlap sequences and order of cyanogen bromide peptides from Mem/72 HA_1. Methionine peptide b was obtained by *Staph. aureus* proteinase digestion of a tryptic peptide.

cleavage after Lys or Arg, as would occur with plasmin, had been expected. The possibility exists therefore, that a small section of polypeptide is removed from HA by the combined action of a proteinase and peptidases, rather than a simple single bond cleavage in the sequence:

$$-\text{Gln-Thr-Gly-Leu-Phe-Gly}$$

$$\text{HA}_1 \xrightarrow{\hspace{3cm}} \xleftarrow{\hspace{5cm}} \text{HA}_2$$

We have also established the order of four of the cyanogen bromide peptides in the overall sequence of HA_1. The major problem here was the presence of three Met-Arg sequences that necessitated blocking the Arg residues with cyclohexa-nedione (Patthy and Smith, 1975) before tryptic cleavage. The sequences of these overlap peptides and the arrangement of the cyanogen bromide peptides are shown in Figure 1. The overlap between CN-1 and CN-2 cannot be confirm-ed until the structure of CN-1 has been established.

When more complete sequence data become available the key chemical differ-ences between successively emerging influenza strains will indicate the mechan-isms behind antigenic shift and drift.

Acknowledgements

We wish to thank Mr. R. W. Cranston and Miss Judith L. Jones for their technical assistance.

REFERENCES

BRIDGEN, P. J. and CROSS, G. A. M. (1976) Nature 263, 613-614.
BUCHER, D. J., LI, S. S-L., KEHOE, J. M. and KILBOURNE, E. D. (1976) Proc. Nat. Acad. Sci. USA. 73, 238-242.
CHOPPIN, P. W. and COMPANS, R. W. (1975) in 'The Influenza Viruses and Influenza' (Ed. Kilbourne, E. D.), pp. 15-51, Academic Press, New York.
CLEGG, J. A. (1974) in 'Parasites in the Immunized Host: Mechanisms of Survival'. Ciba Foundation Symposium 25 (new series), pp. 161-183, Elsevier, Amsterdam.
COMPANS, R. W., KLENK, H-D., CALIGURI, L. A. and CHOPPIN, P. W. (1970) Virology 42, 880-889.
FAZEKAS DE ST. GROTH, S. (1970) Arch. Envirn. Health 21, 293-303.
FAZEKAS DE ST. GROTH, S. (1975) in 'Negative Strand Viruses' (Eds. Mahy, B. W. J. and Barry, R. D.) Vol. 2, pp. 541-554, Academic Press, New York.
FUNATSU, M, FUNATSO, G., ISHIGURU, M., NANNO, S. and HARA, K. (1971) Proc. Jap. Acad. 47, 718-723.
GOTTSCHALK, A. (1969) Nature 222, 452-454.
HARTLEY, B. S. (1970) Biochem. J. 119, 805-822.
INGLIS, A. S. and NICHOLLS, P. W. (1973) J. Chromatog. 79, 344-346.
JACKSON, R. L. and HIRS, C. H. W. (1970) J. Biol. Chem. 245, 624-636.
KILBOURNE, E. D. (1975) Ed. 'The Influenza Viruses and Influenza' Academic Press, New York.

LAVER, W. G. (1971) Virology *45*, 275-288.

LAVER, W. G. and **WEBSTER**, R. G. (1973) Virology *51*, 383-391.

LAVER, W. G. and **WEBSTER**, R. G. (1977) this volume.

LAVER, W. G., **DOWNIE**, J. C. and WEBSTER, R. G. (1974) Virology, *59*, 230-244.

NEUBERGER, A. **GOTTSCHALK**, A., **MARSHALL**, R. D. and SPIRO, R. G. (1972) in 'Glycoproteins' (Ed. Gottschalk, A.) 2nd edition, Part A, pp. 450-490, Elsevier, Amsterdam.

PATTHY, L. and **SMITH**, E. L. (1975) J. Biol. Chem. *250*, 557-564.

PETERSON, J. D., **NEHRLICH**, S., **OYER**, P. E. and STEINER, D. F. (1972) J. Biol. Chem. *247*, 4866-4871.

SCHILD, G. C. and **DOWDLE**, W. R. (1975) in 'The Influenza Viruses and Influenza' (Ed. Kilbourne, E. D.) pp. 316-372, Academic Press, New York.

SCHULZE, I. T. (1970) Virology *42*, 890-904.

SEGREST, J. P. and **JACKSON**, R. L. (1972) Methods Enzymol. *28*, 54-63.

SKEHEL, J. J. (1974) Symposia of the Society for General Microbiology No. **XXIV**. Evolution in the Microbiol. World. pp. 321-343.

SKEHEL, J. J. and **SCHILD**, G. C. (1971) Virology *44*, 396-408.

SKEHEL, J. J. and **WATERFIELD**, M. D. (1975) Proc. Nat. Acad. Sci. USA. *72*, 93-97.

STANLEY, P. M. and **HASLAM**, E. A. (1971) Virology *46*, 764-773.

STANLEY, P. M., **CROOK**, N. E., STREADER, L. G. and DAVIDSON, B. E. (1973) Virology *56*, 640-645.

TOBITA, K. and **KILBOURNE**, E. D. (1975) Arch. Virol. *47*, 367-374.

VIRELIZIER, J-L., **POSTLETHWAITE**, R., SCHILD, G. C. and ALLISON, A. C. (1974) J. Exp. Med. *140*, 1559-1570.

WARD, C. W. and **DOPHEIDE**, T. A. A. (1976) FEBS Letters *65*, 365-368.

WEBSTER, R. G. (1970) Virology *40*, 643-654.

WEBSTER, R. G. and **LAVER**, W. G. (1975) in 'The Influenza Viruses and Influenza' (Ed. Kilbourne, E. D.), pp. 270-314. Academic Press, New York.

WHITE, D. O. (1974) Curr. Top. Microbiol. Immunol. *63*, 1-48.

WILSON, R. J. M. (1974) in 'Parasites in the Immunized Host. Mechanisms of Survival'. Ciba Foundation symposium 25 (New Series). pp. 185-203, Elsevier, Amsterdam.

CHROMATOGRAPHIC SEPARATION AND STRUCTURAL ANALYSIS OF Heq 1 HEMAGGLUTININ

D. J. Bucher and S. S-L. Li

Summary

Amino terminal analysis of the hemagglutinin polypeptides HA_1 and HA_2 were performed on 50-100 mM quantities of protein purified from X-38 influenza vaccine (Heq1N2). A cysteine was identified at position 4 from the amino terminus of HA_1 which had previously been tentatively identified as a serine residue. A chromatographic technique was developed for the separation of the hemagglutinin from nucleoprotein without reduction, thus permitting the disulfides to remain intact for further structural studies of inter and intrachain disulfides.

Cyanogen bromide cleavage was performed on the HA_1 polypeptide. The fragments were separated into six fractions on Sephadex G-50 in 30% formic acid. The original amino terminal fragment was found only in fraction 1, the void volume. Two of the fractions contained at least two sequences and three fractions contained only one amino terminal sequence and were considered to be purified at this step.

We have previously demonstrated that both polypeptides of the influenza viral hemagglutinin can be purified in quantities of 10-30 mg by chromatography on Bio Gel A-5m in the presence of SDS (Bucher *et al.*, 1976). A production lot of an experimental formalin-inactivated influenza vaccine provided the source of viral protein used in these structural studies. The virus in the vaccine was X-38 (Heq1N2) a recombinant resulting from the triparental cross of A/Eng/42/72 (MRC-11)(H3N2), A/PR/8/34 (H0N1) (Ann Arbor variant) and A/equine/ Prague/1/56 (Heq1Neq1) (E. D. Kilbourne, unpublished data). The hemagglutinin (Heq 1) bears little antigenic resemblance to the hemagglutinin of the human A subtype viruses (Kilbourne, 1968) and therefore has been utilized as an 'irrelevant' hemagglutinin in neuraminidase-specific vaccines (Kilbourne *et al.*, 1972; Couch *et al.*, 1974).

This technique of separation of the hemagglutinin polypeptides relies on the fact that asymmetric cleavage of the 75,000 hemagglutinin glycoprotein occurs when influenza virus is propagated *in ovo* (Lazarowitz *et al.*, 1973) yielding HA_1 (50,000) and HA_2 (25,000). Since these polypeptide chains are held together by disulfide bonds, gel chromatography under non-reducing conditions purifies the hemagglutinin away from all viral components with the exception of the nucleoprotein (NP) (Bucher, 1975). Reduction of the HA-NP fraction and reapplication to gel chromatographic columns results in the purification of HA_1 and HA_2 as well as NP. Utilizing vaccine as the starting viral preparation, yields of the hemagglutinin polypeptides average about 50% of the calculated quantity of hemagglutinin protein present (Bucher *et al.*, 1976). This technique has the added advantage that (a) all major viral protein components can be purified in milligram quantities (primarily NP and M) and (b) no proteases are introduced at any point in the purification procedure.

Chromatographic Isolation of the Hemagglutinin Polypeptides and Amino Terminal Analysis of HA_1 and HA_2

The chromatographic isolation of the hemagglutinin polypeptides and their amino terminal analysis have been previously reported (Bucher *et al.*, 1976). Following disruption of 100-300 mg of the viral preparation by heating and sonication in the presence of 10% SDS, the viral preparation is applied to the chromatographic column(s) in a volume of about 10-15 ml. The column separation proceeds on two 2.5 x 90 cm Bio Gel A-5m columns linked in tandem with a flow rate maintained at 12-15 ml/hr. The effluent is monitored at A_{260}. The resultant chromatogram is shown in Figure 1-I. The hemagglutinin-nucleoprotein fraction is recycled to insure separation from the neighboring P and M fractions (Figure 1-II). The large hemagglutinin polypeptide (HA_1) and the small hemagglutinin polypeptide (HA_2) are separated from NP by a third cycle of chromatography after reduction (Figure 1-III). The resultant SDS polyacrylamide gel electrophoresis of the purified NP, HA_1 and HA_2 are shown in Figure 2.

Sodium dodecyl sulfate is removed by anion exchange chromatography and the samples are reduced and alkylated (Bucher *et al.*, 1976). The amino terminal sequence of Heq 1 polypeptides derived from X-38 was determined by automatic Edman degradation with the Beckman sequencer. Ten residues have been identified for HA_1 and 24 for HA_2 (Bucher *et al.*, 1976)

HA$_1$ (Heq 1) $\overset{1}{\text{asp}}$ – lys – ile – $\underset{cys}{\text{ser}}$ – $\overset{5}{\text{leu}}$ – gly – tyr – his – ala – $\overset{10}{\text{val}}$

HA$_2$ (Heq 1) $\overset{1}{\text{gly}}$ – leu – phe – gly – $\overset{5}{\text{ala}}$ – ile – ala – gly

phe – $\overset{10}{\text{ile}}$ – glu – asn – gly – trp – $\overset{15}{\text{glu}}$ –

gly – leu – ile – asp – $\overset{20}{\text{gly}}$ – ? – tyr – gly – tyr

CHROMATOGRAPHIC ISOLATION OF X-38 VACCINE POLYPEPTIDES

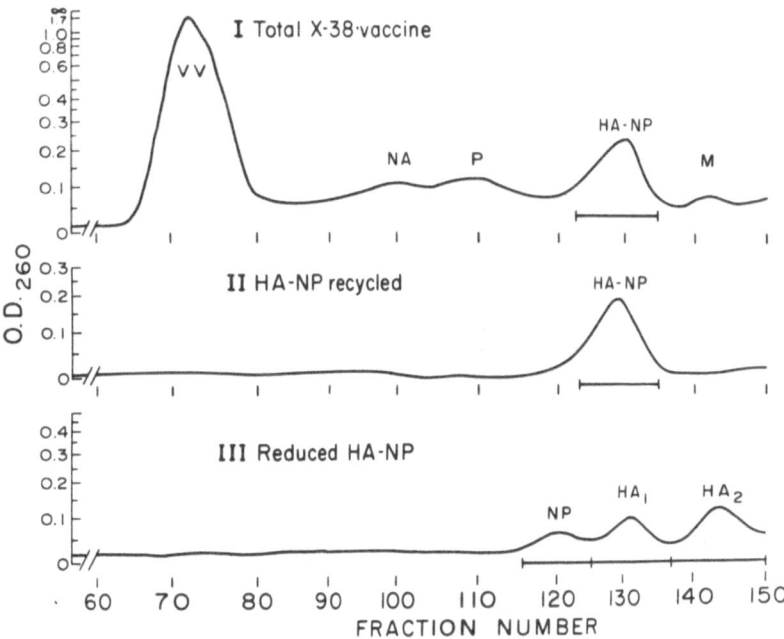

Figure 1

Sodium dodecyl sulfate gel filtration on Bio-Gel A-5m of sodium dodecyl sulfate-disrupted viral vaccine. Chromatograms represent respectively, (1) chromatography of pelleted, disrupted influenza virus vaccine (11) rechromatography of HA-NP fraction, (111) reduction with 0.1 M dithiothreitol and chromatography of HA-NP from 11. Letters designating column fractions: VV, void volume; NA, neuraminidase; P, nonglycosylated polyneptide of molecular weight 122,000; HA-NP, hemagglutinin-nucleoprotein coeluted; M, nonglycosylated polypeptide of 27,000. Elution was performed with 0.02 M Tris-HCl buffer, pH 7.4, containing 0.1% sodium dodecyl sulfate, and 0.05% sodium azide at a flow rate of 12 ml/hr. The total quantity of protein applied was 140 mg. Fractions pooled for viral polypeptides are shown by bars under respective peaks.

The serine identified at position 4 in HA_1 was considered presumptive (Bucher *et al.*, 1976). PTH serine and PTH-S-carboxymethyl-cysteine are not readily distinguishable without radioactive labeling. This residue has now been determined to be a cysteine by radioactive labeling as described below.

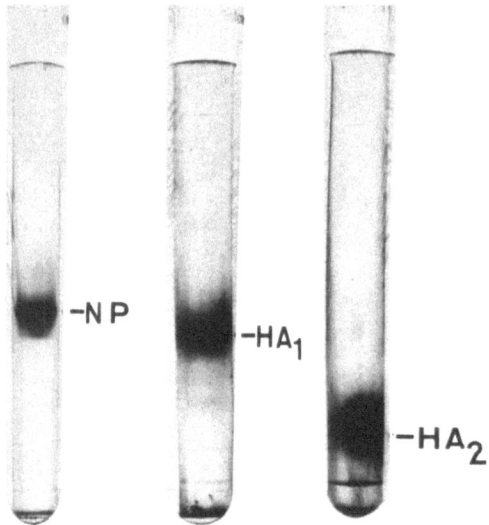

Figure 2

Sodium dodecyl sulfate polyacrylamide gel electrophoresis of NP, HA_1, and HA_2 protein pools from Figure 1, chromatographic cycle 111. Approximately 10-15 μg of viral protein was applied per gel and stained with Coomassie brilliant blue. Viral proteins had been reduced and alkylated for sequence analysis.

In addition we have developed a technique for separation of the hemagglutinin from nucleoprotein without the need to resort to reduction. This method provides us with a source of hemagglutinin with the disulfides intact and will permit localization of both intra- and inter-chain disulfide linkages.

We have also proceeded with the cleavage, separation and amino terminal analysis of cyanogen bromide fragments obtained from HA_1. Cyanogen bromide cleavage of HA_2 was virtually incomplete and will need to be further investigated.

Determination of the position of Cystine-Cysteine Residues by the Use of C^{14} Iodoacetic Acid

The position of cystine/cysteine residues was determined after reduction with dithiothreitol and carboxymethylation with C^{14} iodoacetic acid. Approximately 0.5 mCi of C^{14} iodoacetic acid was added to purified HA_1, followed by the addition of unlabeled iodoacetic acid.(See Bucher *et al.*, 1976). The material was dialyzed for 4 days *versus* distilled water and an additional two days *versus* 20% acetic acid at 4°C. After application to the sequencer and preparation of the resultant phenylthiohydantoins in the usual manner, 0.5 ml ethyl acetate was added to all dried samples and 0.1 ml aliquots used for scintillation counting. A sharp peak of radioactivity was obtained at position 4 (see Figure 3). Therefore the residue at position 4 is a cysteine, not serine.

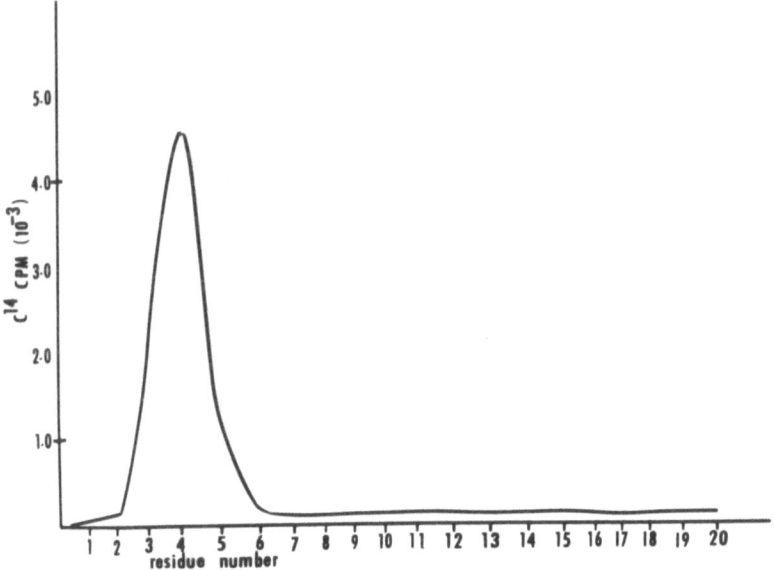

Figure 3

Localization of cys groups from amino terminus by radiolabeling HA_1 with C^{14} iodoacetic acid. Positive identification has been made of a cysteine at residue no. 4.

Separation of the Hemagglutinin Polypeptides without Prior Reduction

Localization of the position of interchain disulfide bonds linking HA_1 and HA_2 as well as intrachain disulfide bonds requires the purification of the hemagglutinin with the disulfide groups intact. According to our present purification technique, the hemagglutinin polypeptides can be separated from NP only after reduction to HA_1 and HA_2. We have thus developed a technique which permits separation of the hemagglutinin from the NP after the fist cycle of SDS gel filtration by chromatography on Bio Gel A-5m in the presence of 6M guanidine hydrochloride

The HA-NP fraction (about 20 mg) is obtained from chromatography on Bio Gel A-5m in 0.1% SDS as described earlier. However, instead of reduction of the polypeptides as generally performed at this point with the separation of HA_1 and HA_2, SDS is removed by chromatography on QAE Sephadex at pH 3 in the presence of 6M urea. The HA-NP fraction with detergent removed is then dialyzed *versus* distilled water for several days to remove the urea.

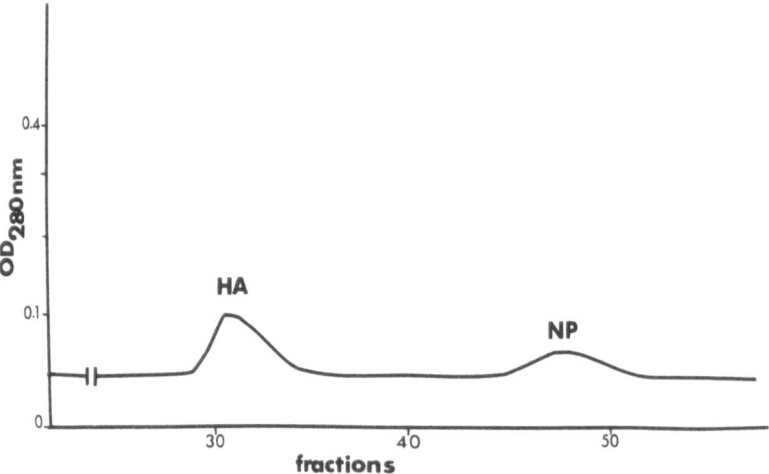

Figure 4

Separation of hemagglutinin from nucleoprotein without reduction by the use of chromatography on Bio-Gel A-5m in 6M guanidine hydrochloride. Column was 1.5 x 90 cm, flow rate was 5 ml/hr.

HA is separated from NP by adjustment of this fraction to 6M guanidine hydrochloride and application to a Bio Gel A-5m column (1.5 x 90 cm). The column is eluted with 6M guanidine hydrochloride. The hemagglutinin is obtained in the void volume (see Figure 4), and the nucleoprotein is eluted at a considerable distance from the hemagglutinin. The products are obtained with considerable purity as can be seen from the SDS gels shown in Figure 5 in which electrophoresis was performed without prior reduction. Evidently the hemagglutinin has aggregated extensively in 6M guanidine hydrochloride thus migrating in the void volume whereas the NP remained in a monomer state. The aggregation of viral glycoproteins in 6M guanidine hydrochloride had previously been reported (McSharry, 1976).

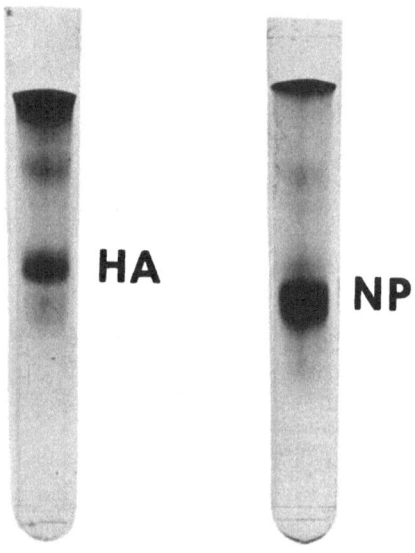

Figure 5

SDS polyacrylamide gel electrophoresis of HA and NP separated as shown in Figure 4. Samples were *not* reduced prior to electrophoresis. Conditions were as reported in Figure 2.

CNBr Cleavage of HA_1 and Separation of Fragments

Purified HA_1 polypeptide was cleaved into smaller fragments utilizing cyanogen bromide and separated by gel filtration. 10 mg of HA_1 was added to 0.5 ml of a solution of 70% formic acid, 0.5 mM DTT containing 20 mg CNBr. The reaction was permitted to continue for 17 hr at room temperature following which the sample was lyophilized. The CNBr fragments of HA_1 were separated by chromatography on a G-50 column (1.5 x 90 cm) in 30% formic acid.

The fragments obtained are shown in Figure 6. Six fractions were obtained with sizes respectively 1) ⟩20,000; 2) 14,000; 3) 7,000; 4) 3,200; 5) 1,6OO; 6) ⟨1,000. The column had previously been calibrated with ovalbumin (43,000) RNase (14,500), insulin B chain (3,300) and insulin A chain (2,300).

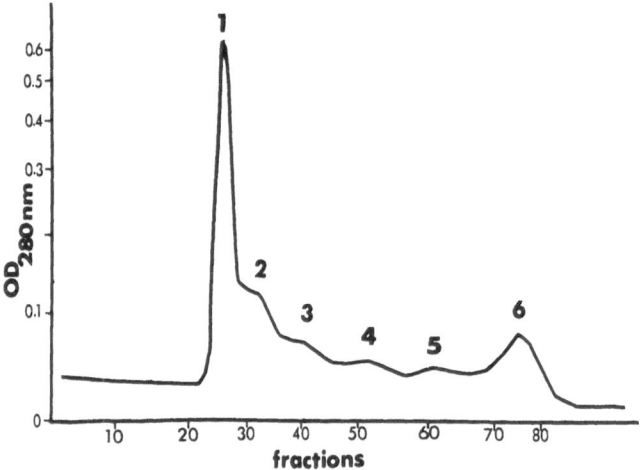

Figure 6

CNBr cleavage of HA_1 (Heq 1) on G-50 Sephadex in 30% formic acid. Column was 1.5 x 90 cm. Flow rate was 25 ml/hr.

Each fraction obtained from the G-50 column was rechromatographed on the same column and lyophilized. The entire sample was used for automatic amino acid sequence analysis with a Beckman sequencer using N,N^1-dimethylallylamine buffer and single acid cleavage (Edman and Begg, 1967; Li *et al.*, 1974; Pisano *et al.*, 1972). Phenylthiohydantoin-amino acids were identified by gas liquid chromatography (Pisano *et al.*, 1972) and thin-layer chromatography (Summers *et al.*, 1973).

Table 1

Fraction	Mol. Wt.	
1	⟩20,000	N-terminal sequence here
2	14,000	at least two sequences
3	7,000	at least two sequences
4	3,200	$\overset{1}{x}$ – phe – val – tyr – $\overset{5}{thr}$ – gly – val – phe – x – $\overset{10}{glu}$
5	1,600	$\overset{1}{leu}$ – ala – val – pro – $\overset{5}{glu}$ – ala – pro – $\overset{8}{ala}$
6	⟨1,000	one sequence

Fractions 4, 5 and 6 produced single amino terminal sequences and evidently were purified completely by chromatography on G-50. Fraction 1, the void volume, contained the amino terminal sequence but appeared fairly heterogeneous. Fractions 2 and 3 both contained at least two sequences. Amino terminal sequences are presented for fragments 4 and 5 in Table 1.

Acknowledgements

The authors wish to express their appreciation to Ms M. Diane Forde and Ms Tatiana Tomko for their expert assistance in this project. The support of Dr. E. D. Kilbourne is gratefully acknowledged. This work was monitored by The Commision on Influenza of the Armed Forces Epidemiological Board and was supported by the U.S. Army Medical Research and Development Command under Research Contract No. DADA 17-69-C-9137.

REFERENCES

BUCHER, D. J., LI, S. S-L., KEHOE, J. M. and KILBOURNE, E. D. (1976) Proc. Nat. Acad. Sci. U.S. *73* , 238-242.

BUCHER, D. J. (1975) in 'Negative Strand Viruses', eds. Mahy, B. W. J. and Barry, R. D. (Academic Press, London) Vol. 1, pp. 133-143.

COUCH, R. B., KASEL, J. A., GERIN, J. L., SCHULMAN, J. L. and KILBOURNE, E. D. (1974) J. Inf. Dis. *129*, 411-420.

EDMAN, P. and BEGG, G. (1967) Eur. J. Biochem. *1* , 80-91.

KILBOURNE, E. D. (1968) Science *160* , 74-76.

KILBOURNE, E. D., SCHULMAN, J. L., COUCH, R. B., and KASEL, J. A. (1972) in 'International Virology 2, Proceedings of the Second International Congress of Virology', ed. Melnick, J. L. (S. Karger, Basel) pp. 118-119.

LAZAROWITZ, S. G., COMPANS, R. W. and CHOPPIN, P. W. (1973) Virology *52*, 199-222.

McSHARRY, J. J. (1976) Abstr. of the Amer. Soc. for Microbiol. p. 231.

PISANO, J., BRONZERT, F. J., and BREWER, H. B. Jr. (1972) Anal. Biochem. *45* , 43-59.

SUMMERS, M. R., SMYTHERS, G. W. and OROSZLAN, S. (1973) Anal. Biochem. *53*, 624-628.

THE PURIFICATION AND STRUCTURAL CHARACTERIZATION OF THE FUSION FACTOR OF SENDAI VIRUS

M. J. Gething, J. M. White, and M. D. Waterfield

Summary

The fusion factor (F) and the hemagglutinin-neuraminidase (HN) of Sendai virus have been purified by lectin affinity chromatography on a *Lens culinaris* (LcH)-Sepharose column. Separation was achieved by sequential elution with two different detergents containing α-methyl mannoside. HN was eluted with the zwitterionic detergent Empigen BB and F with the anionic detergent sodium deoxycholate. F was further purified by molecular sieving on Ultrogel AcA34 and separated into its two component chains (F_1 apparent M.W. 53,000 and F_2 apparent M.W. 15,000) by molecular sieving on Sephadex G-100 after reduction of disulfide bonds. The amino terminus of F_1 was PHE-PHE-GLY-ALA-VAL-ILE-GLY-ILE-ILE-ALA-. This sequence shows identity at six positions with the amino terminal sequence of the small polypeptide chain (HA_2) of the influenza virus hemagglutinin. The amino terminal ten residues of F_1 and HA_2 are extremely hydrophobic and are both generated by proteolytic cleavage of an inactive precursor polypeptide. Structure and function correlations of this cleavage are discussed.

Introduction

Sendai virus has been used for many years to fuse cells, however very little is known about the mechanism of virus induced cell fusion. Recently, studies of virus grown in different types of cells have implicated one of the envelope glycoproteins in the fusion process. Virus grown in L cells or MDBK cells is non-infectious and does not fuse cells whereas virus grown in the allantoic cavity of embryonated fowl eggs is infectious and has fusion activity. Analysis of the proteins of these two types of virus by sodium dodecyl sulfate (SDS) polyacryl-amide gel electrophoresis showed that biological activation is accompanied by proteolytic cleavage of an envelope glycoprotein (F_0) resulting in formation of an active fusion factor, F (Homma and Ohuchi, 1973; Scheid and Choppin, 1974). F has been shown to be composed of two disulfide bonded chains, F_1 and F_2 (Ozawa *et al.*, 1976).

Sendai virus contains a second glycoprotein (HN) which has both hemagglutinating and neuraminidase activities (Tozawa *et al.*, 1973; Scheid and Choppin,
1974). This glycoprotein has not yet been shown to require proteolytic
activation.

In order to study the process of fusion and to characterize membrane proteins
in general the envelope glycoproteins of Sendai virus have been purified and a
preliminary structural characterization of the fusion factor is described.

Materials and Methods

Iodo [^{14}C] acetamide (57 m Ci/mmole) and tritiated potassium borohydride
(3.3 Ci/mmole) were obtained from the Radiochemical Centre, Amersham,
Bucks., U.K.

Virus Growth and Purification

Sendai virus was grown in the allantoic cavity of 10-day-old embryonated
chicken eggs inoculated with 10^4 egg infective doses. Allantoic fluid was harvested after 72 hrs incubation at 37°C and debris was pelleted at 200 x g. The
virus was concentrated by centrifugation at 120,000 x g for 1 hr at 4°C, resuspended in PBS-A and purified by density gradient centrifugation (20-55% sucrose in PBS-A) at 100,000 x g for 2 hrs at 4°C. The visible virus band was collected and concentrated by centrifugation at 120,000 x g for 1 hr at 4°C. The
purified virus was resuspended at 10-20 mg/ml in PBS-A and stored at -70°C.

Tritium Labelling of Sendai Virus Glycoproteins

Sendai virus (10 mg/ml in PBS-A and 2 mM phenylmethylsulphonyl fluoride)
was treated with galactose oxidase (40 units/100 μl in PBS-A) for 1 hr at 20°C.
The virus was centrifuged through 20% sucrose onto a shelf of 55% sucrose.
The virus band was collected and treated with tritiated potassium borohydride
(50 μl in 0.01N NaOH, 5 m Ci, 3.3 Ci/mmole) for 20 min at 20°C. The labelled
virus was centrifuged onto a sucrose shelf as described above and was stored at
-70°C.

Preparation of LcH-Sepharose

Lens culinaris lectin (LcH) was isolated from a commercial sample of orange
lentils by the method of Hayman and Crumpton (1972). Sepharose 4B was
activated with cyanogen bromide (20 mg/ml of settled beads) and coupling of

LcH (1 mg/ml of settled beads) was performed in 0.1 m NaHCO$_3$, pH 8.4 and 0.3 m α-methyl-D-mannoside (Hayman and Crumpton, 1972; Cuatrecasas, 1970) at 4°C for 18 hr.

Separation of F and HN Glycoproteins on LcH-Sepharose

Purified Sendai virions (70 mg) were suspended in 50 ml of 1% Empigen BB, 10 mM Tris-Cl, pH 6.8 and 1 mM phenylmethylsulphonyl fluoride, and sonicated for 30 sec at setting 3 on a Dawe Soniprobe (Type 7530A). The disrupted virions were dialyzed for 16 hr at 4°C against the same buffer and then centrifuged at 120,000 x g for 1 hr at 4°C to pellet nucleocapsids and insoluble M protein. The supernatant containing the solubilized glycoproteins was applied to a column (2.6 x 45 cm) of LcH-Sepharose equilibrated with 1% Empigen BB, pH 5.5. The column was washed with 300 ml of the equilibrating buffer and eluted with 500 ml of 1% Empigen BB, 0.1 M α-methyl-D-mannoside, pH 6.8 and then with 500 ml of 1% sodium deoxycholate, 0.1 M α-methyl-D-mannoside, pH 8.3. The flow rate was 60 ml/hr and 10 ml fractions were collected. The two glycoprotein peaks were pooled separately and concentrated to ~3 ml by ultrafiltration through a PM-10 membrane in an Amicon Diaflo apparatus.

Purification of F on Ultrogel AcA34

The partly purified F glycoprotein (3 ml, 1.3 mg/ml) was applied to a column of Ultrogel AcA34 (1.6 cm x 2 m) equilibrated with 1% sodium deoxycholate, pH 8.3 and the column was eluted at 10 ml/hr. Fractions of 2 ml were collected and aliquots were analyzed by electrophoresis on SDS-acrylamide gels. The fractions containing pure F protein were pooled and concentrated to 2 ml by ultrafiltration through a PM-10 membrane in an Amicon Diaflo. Deoxycholate was removed by dialysis for 4 days against 0.5% pyridine, pH 8.5.

Reduction and Alkylation of F

Pure F glycoprotein (3 mg) in 3 ml of 6 M guanidine hydrochloride, 0.1 M Tris, pH 8.3 was treated with 1 mM dithiothreitol for 2 hr at 37°C. Iodo[^{14}C]acetamide (10 μmole, 5.7 m Ci/mole) was then added and the mixture incubated for 1 hr at 37°C. Excess iodoacetamide was reacted with 2-mercaptoethanol (150 μmole) and the solution was dialyzed for 16 hr against 500 ml of 6 M formic acid. The alkylated sample was then applied to a column of Sephadex G-100 (2.6 x 90 cm) equilibrated with 6 M urea, 0.2 M formic acid. The column was eluted at 10 ml/hr and 2 ml fractions were collected. F_1 and F_2 peaks were pooled separately and dialyzed against 0.5% pyridine, pH 8.5 and concentrated by lyphilization.

Hemagglutination Assay

Aliquots of 0.025 ml of 2-fold serial dilutions of viral protein samples in PBS-A were mixed with 0.025 ml of 1% chicken red cells in PBS-A. The HA titer is expressed as the reciprocal of the final dilution which agglutinated the red cells after 2 hrs incubation at 4°C.

Neuraminidase Assay

An aliquot of viral protein was mixed with 0.1 ml of 0.2 M sodium acetate buffer, pH 5.0. 0.1 ml of fetuin (10 mg/ml) was added as substrate and the mixture was incubated at 37°C for 6 min. Liberated N-acetyl neuraminic acid was assayed by the 2-thiobarbituric acid method (Aminoff, 1961).

Amino Acid Sequence Analysis

Amino terminal sequences were determined using a Beckman 890C Sequencer and the 0.1 M Quadrol program of Brauer *et al*. (1975). PTH amino acids were identified by high pressure liquid chromatography (HPLC) using a Waters HPLC and a μ Bondapak C18 column. Assignments of amino acids were confirmed by back hydrolysis of PTH amino acids in hydroiodic acid (Smithies *et al*., 1971) followed by amino acid analysis on a Durrum D500 amino acid analyser, and by gas chromatographic analysis by the techniques of Pisano *et al*. (1969).

Results

Tritium Labelling of Virion Glycoproteins

Analysis of Sendai viral proteins by Coomassie Blue staining after SDS-poly-acrylamide gel electrophoresis (Figure 1) reveals five major bands corresponding to the polymerase (P), hemagglutinin-neuraminidase (HN), nucleocapsid protein (NC), the larger polypeptide component of the fusion factor (F_1) and the matrix protein (M). Autoradiography of a similar gel of virus which has been labelled with tritium on galactose residues using the galactose oxidase-tritiated borohydride method (Critchley, 1974) shows four distinct carbohydrate containing bands (Figure 1). One of these bands runs with the bromophenol blue marker near the bottom of the gel and may be glycolipid. The remaining radioactivity is found in the HN protein (apparent M.W. 69,000) and in the two component chains of the fusion factor which have apparent molecular weights of 53,000 (F_1) and 15,000 (F_2). It can be seen that F_1 and F_2 are equally labelled with this technique although F_2 stains very weakly with Coomassie Blue. These results suggest that a considerable part of the carbohydrate on the fusion factor is confined to a small region of the polypeptide backbone. Furthermore, the ability to radioactively label F_2 makes it possible to monitor the purification of this polypeptide.

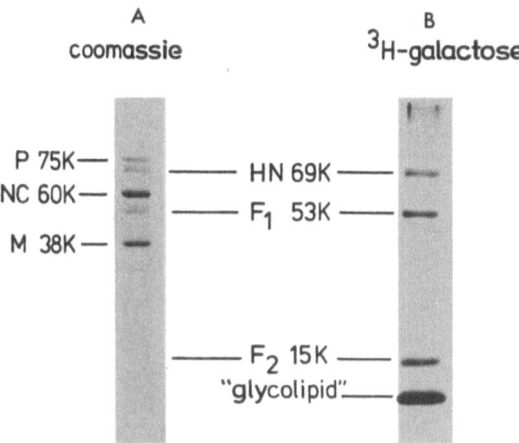

Figure 1

Polyacrylamide gel electrophoresis of the polypeptides of Sendai virus grown in embryonated fowl eggs.

A   stained with Coomassie Brilliant Blue;

B   autoradiograph of a gel of virus labelled with $^3[H]$-borohydride by the galactose oxidase method. The origin is at the top.

Separation of Sendai Glycoproteins on LcH-Sepharose

Sendai virus (30-70 mg) labelled with tritium on galactose residues was disrupted with the zwitterionic detergent Empigen BB (uncharged between pH 3-10) and the solution was centrifuged to remove nucleocapsids and the M protein which precipitates from solution at low ionic strength. The supernatant was chromatographed on a column of LcH-Sepharose and the column effluent was monitored for protein (A_{280}), tritium label, hemagglutinating and neuraminidase activities (Figure 2). Samples from the peak fractions were analyzed on SDS-polyacrylamide gels (Figure 3). The F and HN glycoproteins were bound to the column while the peak of unretarded material contained some nucleocapsid protein and polymerase. The column was developed with 0.1 M α-methyl-D-mannoside in 1% Empigen BB, pH 6.8 which resulted in the elution of a small peak of 'glycolipid' followed by a protein containing peak consisting of HN and a small amount of F. The majority of the F protein was eluted when the column was washed with 0.1 M α-methyl-D-mannoside in 1% sodium deoxycholate, pH 8.3. Thus this procedure resulted in the separation and purification of the two glycoproteins of Sendai virus.

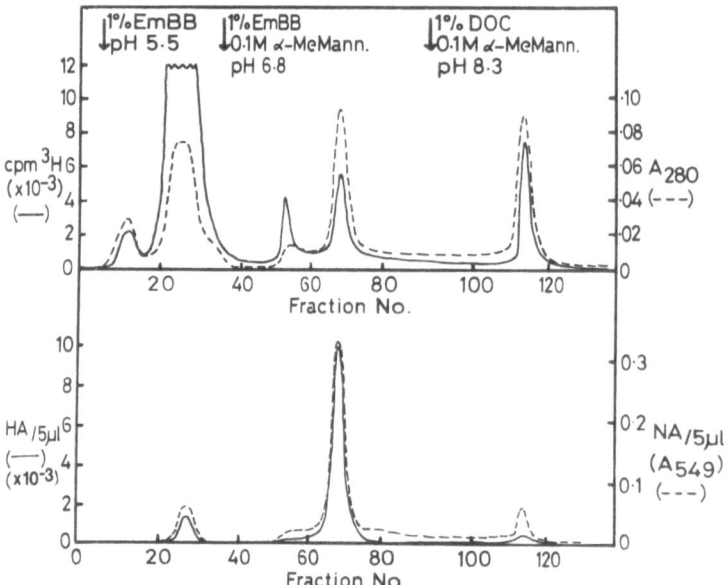

Figure 2

Fractionation of Sendai virus glycoproteins by affinity chromatography on LcH-Sepharose. The details are described in Methods. 50 μl aliquots were analyzed for radioactivity and 5 μl aliquots for hemagglutinin and neuraminidase activity. Polyacrylamide gel analysis of the peak fractions is shown in Figure 3.

Purification of F on Ultrogel AcA34

The fractions containing F from the LcH-Sepharose column were pooled and chromatographed on Ultrogel AcA34 in 1% sodium deoxycholate, pH 8.3. A single asymmetric peak of protein was eluted from the column (Figure 4). Fractions across the peak were analyzed by SDS-polyacrylamide gel electrophoresis (Figure 4, inset). This showed that the main portion of the peak contained pure F glycoprotein, while the trailing edge contained a small amount of HN. Fractions containing pure F were pooled and concentrated. The yield of F was 50-80% of theoretical.

Separation of F_1 and F_2 on Sephadex G-100 after Reduction and Alkylation of F

The purified F glycoprotein was separated from sodium deoxycholate by dialysis, treated with dithiothreitol to reduce sulphdryl groups and reacted with

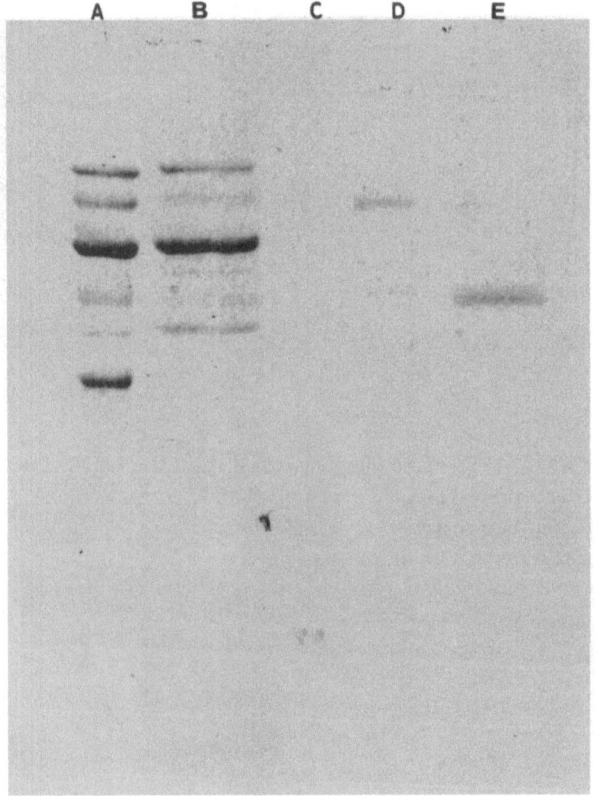

Figure 3

Polyacrylamide gel electrophoresis of the peak fractions obtained on affinity chromatography
of Sendai virus glycoproteins on LcH-Sepharose.
A, Whole virus; B, fraction 24 (100 μl aliquot); C, fraction 52 (25 μl); D, fraction 69 (25 μl);
E, fraction 112 (25 μl). The origin is at the top of the figure.

iodo[^{14}C]acetamide. Chromatography of the alkylated protein on Sephadex
G-100 resulted in the separation of the F_1 and F_2 component polypeptide
chains (Figure 5).

Sequence Analysis of F, F_1 and F_2

Analysis of F in the sequencer revealed a single amino terminal sequence which
is shown in Table 1. Since F contains two disulfide bonded polypeptide chains
F_1 and F_2 this result suggested that one chain had a blocked amino terminus
which was not reactive with the Edman reagent phenylisothiocyanate.

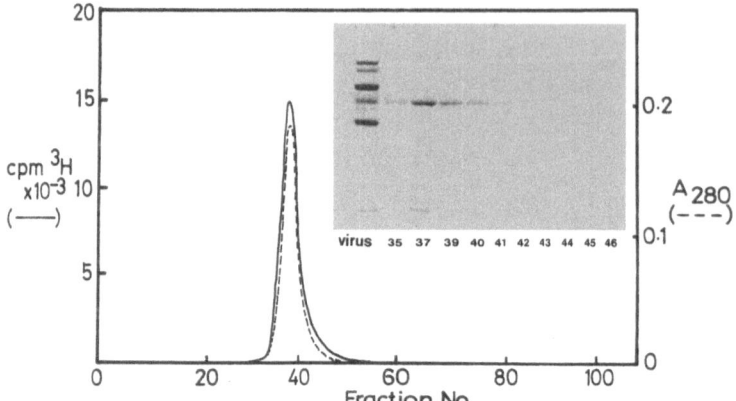

Figure 4

Chromatography of F on Ultrogel AcA34. **The fractions containing F from the LcH-Sepharose
column (Figure 2) were pooled, concentrated and chromatographed on Ultrogel AcA34. The
details are described in Methods. 50 μl aliquots were analyzed for radioactivity. A polyacrylamide gel analysis of the peak fractions is shown in the inset.**

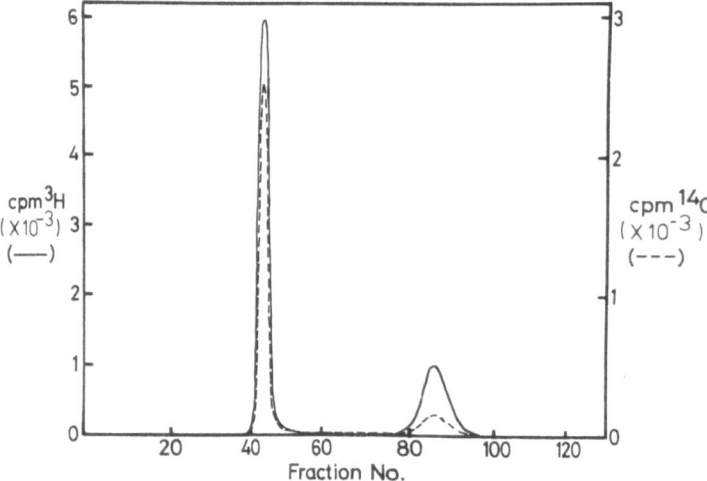

Figure 5

Separation of F_1 and F_2 polypeptides on Sephadex G-100 after reduction and alkylation of
F. The details are described in Methods. 100 μl aliquots were analyzed for radioactivity.

Sequence analysis of the individual component chains confirmed that the
blocked amino terminus was present on F_2 while the amino terminal sequence
determined on whole F was present on F_1.

Table 1

Amino Terminal Sequence of F_1 Chain of Sendai Virus Fusion Factor

NH_2–Phe–Phe–Gly–Ala–Val–Ile–Gly–Ile–Ile–Ala–.

Discussion

Purification of the glycoproteins from Sendai virus on a scale sufficient for structural study has been achieved by affinity chromatography on lentil agglutinin-Sepharose in detergents. Separation of the 2 glycoproteins F and HN was achieved by using two different detergents. The virus was disrupted in the zwitterionic detergent Empigen BB which is uncharged at the pH used for chromatography on lentil-Sepharose. The HN was eluted by α-methyl-D-mannoside in Empigen BB and F was eluted with α-methyl-D-mannoside in deoxycholate. The ability to use 2 different detergents to achieve separation may result from differences in hydrophobicity of the two glycoproteins, however the basis for the separation has not been determined. Previous methods of separation have taken advantage of molecular weight differences or the binding of the HN protein to the sialylated substrate fetuin (Scheid and Choppin, 1974). These techniques have been used on the radiochemical level and have proved difficult to apply to milligram amounts of protein. The advantage of the techniques used in this study is that sufficient protein can be purified for structural characterization by conventional techniques. In the present study F and HN were radioactively labelled on their carbohydrate side chains by oxidation with galactose oxidase and reduction with ^{3}H-borohydride. This procedure made it possible to monitor the glycoproteins during purification. In addition the use of non-denaturing detergents made it possible to follow neuraminidase and hemagglutinin activities. The final purification of F was achieved by molecular sieving on Ultrogel and F_1 and F_2 were separated after reduction and alkylation of disulfide bonds with ^{14}C-iodoacetamide and molecular sieving on Sephadex G-100 in urea. By this technique a second radioactive label, on cysteine residues, was introduced into the polypeptides. These results confirm that F is made up of two polypeptide chains which differ considerably in apparent molecular weight – F_1 of 53,000 daltons and F_2 of 15,000 daltons. Since both chains are glycosylated as shown by the distribution of ^{3}H-galactose residues, these molecular weights could be considerably overestimated. It is clear that a large proportion of the galactose accessible to galactose oxidase is present in a limited region of the polypeptide backbone since F_2 contains at least as much radio-activity as F_1. It has been shown previously that F is generated by proteolytic cleavage of F_0 (Homma and Ohuchi, 1973; Scheid and Choppin, 1974). Sequence analysis of F shows that the N-terminus of the smaller polypeptide chain component, F_2, is blocked while the larger component F_1 has a free amino terminus. These results suggest that the order of biosynthesis is NH_2-F_2-F_1-COOH. The orientation of F in the membrane of the virus is not known. However by analogy with the structure of the hemagglutinin of influenza virus (Waterfield *et al.*, 1977), from studies of other membrane proteins such as gly-cophorin (Tomita and Marchesi, 1975) and from current concepts on the bio-synthesis of membrane proteins (Blobel, 1975) we suggest a model for the acti-vation of F which is outlined in Figure 6.

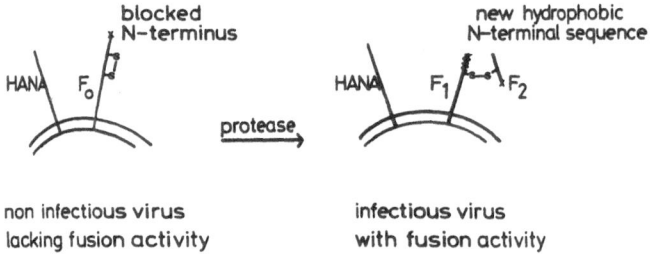

Figure 6

Diagrammatic representation of the protease activation of Sendai virus fusion factor.

Cleavage of F_0 to F which is made up of F_1 disulfide bonded to F_2 results in the generation of an amino terminal hydrophobic region on F_1 (Table 1). When this region is compared with hydrophobic regions of other proteins (Segrest and Feldmann, 1975) it falls into a group of extremely hydrophobic sequences, some of which are found in lipid associated polypeptides. This observation suggests that the hydrophobic amino terminus of F_1 may play a role in inter-action with the host cell membrane during infection by the virus and during cell fusion. However there is no experimental basis for these speculations.

The overall features of the protease activation of Sendai virus infectivity and fusion activity have several features in common with the protease activation of influenza virus infectivity. In both viruses a precursor to the glycoprotein – F or HA – is cleaved with the appearance of biological activity. In each case cleavage results in the generation of an amino terminal hydrophobic sequence which shows 6 out of 10 identities in the first 10 amino acid residues.

The precise definition of the cleavage reaction must await structural analysis of the precursor polypeptides since a portion of the polypeptide chain may be removed during cleavage. Structural similarities between the HA of influenza and the fusion factor of Sendai suggest similarities in function. However the precise understanding of the function of these polypeptides must await further studies of structure and biology.

REFERENCES

AMINOFF, D. (1961) Biochem. J. *81*, 384-392.
BLOBEL, G. and DOBBERSTEIN. B. (1975) J. Cell. Biol. *67*. 835-851.
BRAUER, A. W., MARGOLIES, M. N. and HABER, E. (1975) Biochemistry *14*, 3029-3035.
CRITCHLEY, D. R. (1974) Cell *3*, 121-125.
CUATRECASAS, P. (1970) J. Biol. Chem. *245*, 3059-3065.
HOMMA, M and OHUCHI, M (1973) J. Virol. *12*, 1457-1465.
OZAWA, M., ASANO, A. and OKADA, Y. (1976) Febs Lett. *70*, 145-149.
PISANO, J. J. and BRONZERT, T. J. (1969) J. Biol. Chem. *244*, 5597-5607.
SEGREST, J. P. and FELDMANN, R. J. (1974) J. Mol. Biol. *87*, 853-858.
SCHEID, A. and CHOPPIN, P. W. (1974) Virology *57*, 475-490.
SCHEID, A. and CHOPPIN, P. W. (1976) Virology *69*, 265-277.
SMITHIES, O., GILSON, D., FANNING, E. M., GOODFLEISH, R. M., GILMAN, J. G. and BALLANTYNE, D. C. (1971) Biochemistry *10*, 4912-4921.
TOMITA, M. and MARCHESI, V. T. (1975) Proc. Nat. Acad. Sci. USA. *72*, 2964-2968.
TOZAWA, H., WATANABE, M. and ISHIDA, N. (1973) Virology *55*, 242-253.
WATERFIELD, M. D., SKEHEL, J. J., NAKASHIMA, Y., GURNETT, A. and BILHAM, T. (1977) this volume.

THE CHEMISTRY OF ANTIGENIC DETERMINANTS ON PROTEIN MOLECULES

Ruth Arnon

Introduction

In the course of an immune response, antigens exhibit two distinct reactivities, which may not necessarily coincide. The first is the *immunogenicity*, namely the capacity of the antigenic substance to elicit an immune response, and the second is the *antigenic specificity*, which refers to their capacity to interact, in a specific manner, with antibodies or with immune lymphocytes, regardless of how these have been raised. The region in the antigenic molecule which directly comes into contact with the active site of the antibodies, or with a cell surface receptor is defined as an *antigenic determinant*. Proteins and large polypeptides may carry a large number and variety of possible antigenic determinants which determine the antigenic specificity of that particular macromolecule.

In order to investigate the contribution of the various structural parameters to the antigenic properties of proteins there are two main approaches: the first uses as a starting material an immunogenic protein, which is subjected to enzymatic or chemical degradation. The resulting fragments are subsequently screened for their capacity to elicit an immune response, or to interact with antibodies induced by the original protein. In that manner information is obtained about size and nature of fragments which possess antigenic properties. This approach to the elucidation of the molecular requirements for antigenicity may be termed analytical, as it is based on the dismembering of a natural antigen. An alternative approach is the synthetic one, according to which the starting materials are the small building blocks of proteins, namely amino acids, which by themselves have no antigenic properties whatsoever. They are used for the synthesis of macromolecular polypeptides, which are investigated for their immunogenicity or antigenicity. The synthetic approach offers the advantage that, once the antigenicity of one synthetic material has been unequivocally demonstrated, dozens of analogs of it may be prepared and tested. Since the chemistry of these compounds is known, it should be feasible, through a systematic study of such polymers, which show only limited controlled variations in their chemical formulae and structure, to arrive at conclusions concerning the role of various structural features in their antigenic function. The antigenic complexity of proteins stems both from their primary structure and from the three dimensional folding of their polypeptide chain(s). Studies on the antigenic properites of naturally occurring proteins included therefore the elucidation of the role of various molecular parameters in the antigenic functions, as well as an attempt to identify specific residues which are crucial in the antigenic determinants. Information in this direction is usually obtained either by chemical modification of particular amino acid residues and analysis of its effect on the antigenic properties, or by studying the immunological cross-reaction between homologous proteins. When detailed information is available on sequence and structure of such related proteins, it may be possible to localize and identify some antigenic determinants.

A combination of the various approaches outlined above, using both natural and synthetic materials, has contributed to our understanding of the chemistry of antigenic determinants of proteins, as will be illustrated in the following.

Synthetic Polypeptide Antigens

Until 1960 only natural materials were known to be antigenic. At that time it has been shown that homo-oligomers of amino acid could enhance the antigenicity of a poorly immunogenic protein, gelatin (Sela and Arnon, 1960a, 1960b; Arnon and Sela, 1960). A subsequent detailed investigation of the immunochemical properties of many polypeptidyl gelatins, which indicated that the best potentiator of the immune response in a specific manner was an oligopeptide containing either only tyrosine or both tyrosine and glutamic acid, led to the preparation of a completely synthetic antigen. This was a multichain, or branched, synthetic polypeptide, in which poly-*DL*-alanine side chains were attached to the ε-amino groups of a poly-*L*-lysine backbone, and the polyalanyl chains were in turn elongated with peptides containing *L*-tyrosine and *L*-glutamic acid (Sela and Arnon, 1960c; Sela *et al.*, 1962). This polymer was denoted (T,G)-A- -L, and it provoked the formation of antibodies specific for the peptides of tyrosine and glutamic acid (the (T,G) determinant).

Following the synthesis of this first antigenic material, many analogs have been prepared and tested. Knowing the chemistry of these compounds it seemed possible, through a study of copolymers showing only limited variations in their chemical formulae, to arrive at conclusions concerning the role of various structural features in their antigenic function. The problems considered over the years included the role of shape, size, composition and electrical charge of the macromolecule; of the locus in the molecule of the area important for immunogenicity, as well as the optical configuration of its component amino acids and the steric conformation of the immunogenic macromolecule. The results may be summarized as follows:

Homopolymers of amino acids are usually very poor immunogens, but the immunogenicity increases with increased variations in composition. While macromolecular substances are more reliably immunogenic, low molecular weight peptide conjugates may still be immunogenic, provided they have the right composition (de Weck, 1974). The presence of electrical charges on a macromolecule is not a minimal requirement for it to be immunogenic, but it affects the antigenic specificity (Fuchs and Sela, 1963). Moreover, when the antigen is charged, an inverse relationship exists between the net electrical charge of the immunogen and that of the antibodies it provokes (Sela and Mozes, 1966).

Peptides of opposite optical configuration are exquisitely distinguished by specific antibodies, which are usually stereospecific, i.e., totally unreactive towards the other optical isomer; but, polymers containing exclusively D-amino acids are poor immunogens and easily induce immunological tolerance, unless administered in very small doses. It seems that the inefficient formation of antibodies to polymers of D-amino acids in cases of tolerance is due to their slow and incomplete catabolism.

One of the crucial factors that affect the antigenic properties of the molecule is the accessibility of the antigenic determinants (Sela et al., 1962). The importance of the specific location of the determinant on the synthetic polymer was studied by comparing the response to the above mentioned synthetic antigen, (T,G)-A--L, with that elicited by an antigen very similar to it in composition, but in which the (T,G) peptide were directly attached to the ε-amino groups of the polylysyl backbone, and were subsequently elongated at their terminal positions with poly-DL-alanine chains (Fig. 1). The latter polymer, though of the same amino acid composition as (T,G)-A--L, does not possess its immuno-

228

genicity, nor the antigenic specificity of the (T,G) group. Thus, by changing the locus of the functional antigenic group it is possible to render a macromolecule either antigenic or non-antigenic, and the conclusion is that the antigenic determinant cannot be hidden in the interior of the molecule but must be exposed or accessible in order to exert its effect.

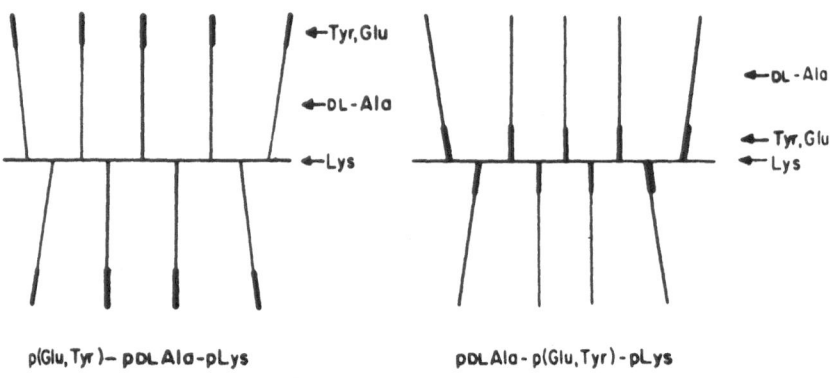

p(Glu,Tyr)– pᴅʟAlα-pLys   pᴅʟAlα- p(Glu,Tyr)-pLys

Figure 1

Schematic representation of multichain copolymer in which *L*-tyrosine and *L*-glutamic acid residues are attached to multi-poly- *DL*-alanyl-poly- *L*-lysine, ((T,G)-A- -L), and of one in which tyrosine and glutamic acid are attached directly to the lysine backbone and then alongated with alanine peptides. (A-(T,G)- -L).

A very interesting factor in the chemistry of antigenic determinants of protein is the role of the composition and structure of the determinant itself. This question was approached by the study of synthetic antigens containing peptides with ordered sequence; such antigens enable the detailed analysis of simple antigenic determinants. For example, in the synthetic antigen (T,G)-A- -L, the determinant is a random oligopeptide containing tyrosine and glutamic acid. In a systematic study using a series of defined tetrapeptides, each composed of tyrosine and glutamic acid, attached to multichain poly-*DL*-alanine carrier, it was possible to demonstrate that the main antigenic determinant in the randomly polymerized (T,G)-A- -L is the peptide with the sequence of Tyr-Tyr-Glu-Glu (T-T-G-G). The random and the ordered antigens exhibited similar antigenic specificity and were found to be under the same genetic control. A similar determinant, T-G-T-G, hooked on the polymeric carrier, yielded a material which, although immunogenic by itself, showed almost no cross-reactivity with antibodies to the random polymer (Mozes *et al.*, 1974). Thus, these two peptides T-T-G-G, and T-G-T-G, which differ from each other only in the exchange of position of two residues, confer completely different immunological properties on the macromolecular antigen they are part of.

An important conclusion obtained from the study of synthetic antigens concerns the crucial role that spatial conformation plays in the antigenic properties of protein molecules. Since this parameter is one of the most influencial in immunochemistry it will be dealt with in more detail.

Role of Conformation in Antigenicity

The decisive role of conformation in determining the antigenic specificity of protein and polypeptide antigens is a widely recognized phenomenon, and was discussed in detail in several recent reviews (Crumpton, 1974; Arnon, in press). A large body of experimental evidence indicates that a drastic change of the antigenic properties occurs upon denaturation of native proteins (by heat or chemical modification) or upon unfolding of their polypeptide chains. The denatured or unfolded proteins are usually still immunogenic, but their antigenic specificity is totally different from that of the corresponding native proteins.

In many instances more subtle conformational alterations in a protein were also accompanied by a change in antigenic reactivity. The best example of such systems concerns the change in the antigenicity associated with the removal of the haem group from sperm whale myoglobin: in the conversion of metmyoglobin to apomyoglobin the loss of haem is associated with only small structural change, and in parallel, the antigenic properties of the two molecular species are not much different. However, the precipitate formed between metmyoglobin and anti-apomyoglobin was shown to be colorless and did not contain the ferrihaem group (Crumpton and Wilkinson, 1966), indicating that the antibodies specific toward the haem-free molecule, not only recognized the small structural differences, but also induced a conformational change in the metmyoglobin and released the haem group from it during the antigen-antibody interaction.

For a better assessment of the contribution of spatial conformation to the antigenic properties of a protein molecule, one should first analyze the various structural features which affect the antigenic specificity. Antibodies elicited in response to immunization with protein antigens are reactive with various antigenic determinants, and may be directed against one or more of the structural aspects of the protein. These consist of the primary structure (the amino acid sequence of the polypeptide chain), the secondary structure (which is dictated by the backbone of the polypeptide, such as α-helix and β-pleated sheet), the tertiary structure (which is conferred by interactions between various groupings in the chain and is associated with its folding), and the quaternary structure (which results from specific association of several polypeptide chains to form a multisubunit protein). The antigenic determinants were, therefore, divided on a theoretical basis into two broad categories 'sequential' and 'conformational' (Sela et al., 1967), depending on whether their specificity is due only to stretches of amino acid sequences in the protein, or to the other structural features mentioned above.

According to this classification a sequential determinant was defined as one due to a segment in the amino acid sequence in its unfolded or linear conformation, and antibodies to such a determinant are expected to react with a peptide of identical or similar sequence. On the other hand, a conformational determinant was defined as one resulting from the steric conformation of the antigenic macromolecule, and leading to antibodies which would not necessarily react with peptides derived from that area of the molecule. Thus conformational determinants would include those determinants composed of amino acid residues that are remote in the unfolded peptide chain(s) but occupy juxtapositions in the native folded structure.

Examination of the three dimensional structures of a number of globular proteins reveals that they contain short sequences of adjacent amino acids whose side chains are partially or fully exposed on the surface of the protein, e.g., residues 77-80 and 81-85 in sperm whale myoglobin (Dickerson, 1964), and residues 53-63 of lamprey hemoglobin. Consequently, the existence of sequential determinants in globular proteins is at least theoretically feasible. However, in practice, little convincing evidence in support of their occurrence has been reported. In cases where short peptide fragments of a protein were shown to interfere with the interaction of the native protein with its antibodies, this capacity is often due to the fact that the peptides are induced by the antibodies to refold into the structure that they assume in the native protein. There are only a few, clear-cut cases where sequential determinants can be demonstrated, such as the terminal segments of collagen (Becker et al., 1972) or fragments of silk fibroin (Cebra, 1961) but, in general, antibodies to native proteins are directed mostly, and in several cases exclusively, against conformation-dependent determinants.

In sperm whale myoglobin, for example, even though the molecule lacks any disulfide bonds to stabilize its structure, the antigenic regions of the molecule were shown to occupy 'corners' in the folded structure (Atassi, 1975), as shown in Figure 2. A space filling molecular model reveals that these corners coincide with the more exposed areas, which due to the folding of the polypeptide chain are held in a fixed conformation. Moreover, as mentioned earlier, the haem group which is non-covalently bound to the protein moiety, and can be removed to yield the haem-free protein (apomyoglobin), also contributes to the antigenic properties (Crumpton and Wilkinson, 1966). In lysozyme at least two well-defined antigenic determinants were characterized, the one containing an intra-chain disulfide bridge (Arnon and Sela, 1969) and the other – an interchain disulfide linking the amino and carboxyl terminal regions (Fujio *et al.*, 1968a). and both were shown to be strictly conformation-dependent.

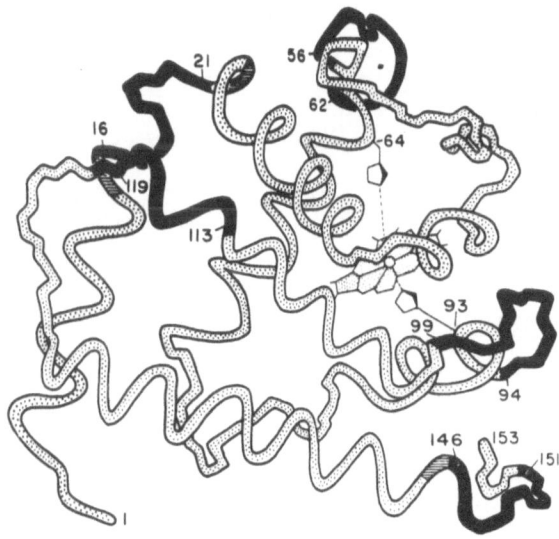

Figure 2

A schematic diagram showing the mode of folding of myoglobin and its antigenic structure. The solid black portions represent segments which have been shown to comprise accurately entire antigenic determinants. The striped parts, each corresponding to one amino acid residue only, can be part of antigenic site with some antisera. The dotted portions represent areas which have been shown exhaustively to reside outside antigenically reactive regions. (From Atassi, 1975)

In view of the role played by conformation in determining antigenicity, it is not surprising that antigenic cross-reactivity has been proposed as a sensitive probe for conformational differences and similarities between related proteins. However, whereas cross-reactivity could be taken as an indication for similarity, the lack of cross-reactivity does not necessarily imply gross differences in conformation. For example, native hen egg-white lysozyme and bovine α-lactalbumin which share 40% of their amino acid sequence (Brew *et al.*, 1969), do not cross-react (Arnon and Maron, 1970), but as shown in Figure 3, their unfolded poly-

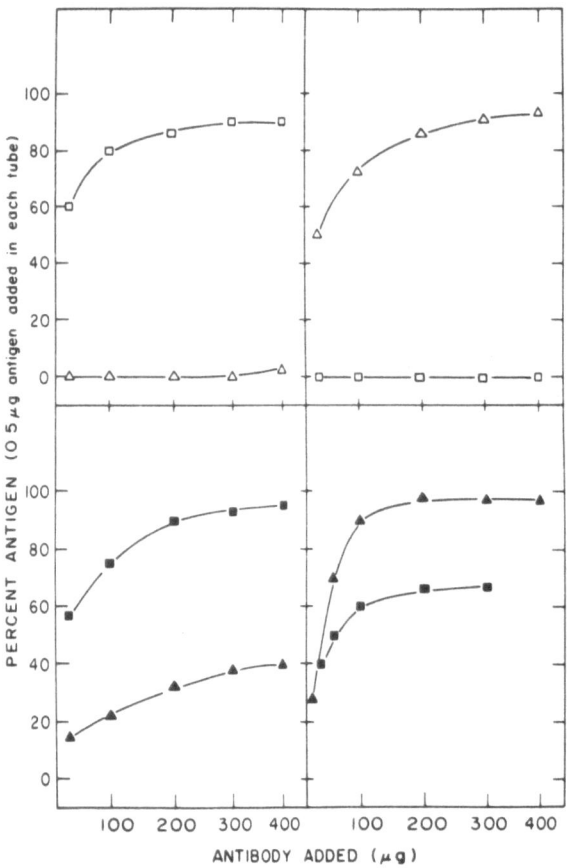

Figure 3

Antigen binding capacity of native and open-chain egg-white lysozyme and bovine α-lactalbumin, by isolated antibodies against native lysozyme (upper left), native lactalbumin (upper right), RCM lysozyme (lower left) and RCM lactalbumin (lower right). The antigens are: □, native lysozyme; △, native lactalbumin; ■, RCM lysozyme; ▲, RCM lactalbumin.

peptide chains show marked cross-reaction (Arnon and Maron, 1971). These results reveal obvious differences between the 'hydrophilic peripheries' of the proteins, in spite of possible similarities in their main chain conformation.

The role of conformation in antigenic specificity was most convincingly demonstrated by the use of two synthetic antigens, both containing the same tyrosyl-alanyl-glutamyl sequence (Fig. 4). The first one was a high molecular weight ordered copolymer composed of the repeated sequence of the tripeptide Tyr-Ala-Glu, which had been previously shown to exist as a α-helix. In the second antigen the same tripeptide was attached to a branched polymer of alanine, and there it exists as a random coil. These two polymers elicited the formation of antibodies with distinct specificities, and no cross-reaction occurred between them (Schechter et al., 1971). Furthermore, the system of the branched polymer was efficiently inhibited by the tripeptide, whereas the system of the helical peptide was not. Inhibition of the latter system was achieved only with oligopeptides of the general formula $(\text{Tÿr-Ala-Glu})_n$, which, as such, possess very low helical structure, but are converted into α-helix upon interaction with the antibody to the helical polymer. It was, therefore, concluded that the antigenicity of the α-helical copolymer is conformation-dependent. Structural conformation is thus an important factor in the array of molecular parameters affecting antigenicity.

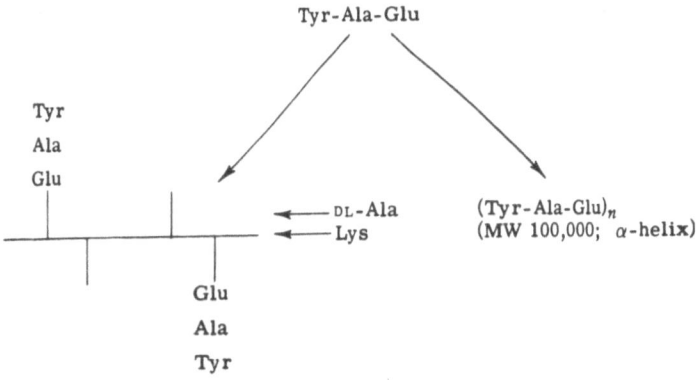

(MW 75,000; multichain)

Figure 4

Synthetic branched polymer in which peptides of sequence Tyr-Ala-Glu are attached to the amino termini of polymeric side chains in multi-poly- *DL* -alanyl-poly- *L* -lysine (left) and a periodic polymer of the tripeptide Tyr-Ala-Glu (right).

234

Defined Antigenic Determinants in Proteins

As mentioned in the beginning, the approach most commonly used for the identification of antigenicall reactive regions of proteins is their fragmentation by chemical cleavage or limited proteolysis, and the screening of the resultant fragments for immunologically active components. This approach, in spite of its shortcomings, led to informative results ever since the early experiments in 1957 by Lapresle and by Porter with serum albumins (Porter, 1957; Lapresle and Darieux, 1957).

When the approach is employed on unfolded proteins, the resulting fragments will usually contain sequential determinants. In that manner information was obtained on antigenic structure of oxidized ribonuclease (ribox), reduced lysozyme or oxidized ferredoxin (Arnon, in press). Sequential determinants were revealed also in folded proteins, in areas of loose structure, such as the non-helical N- and C-terminal regions of the collagen molecule (Becker *et al.*, 1972). These are the molecular regions in which most of the interspecies differences are manifested, and they contribute appreciably to the antigenic specificity of collagen. In some cases these determinants, whose specificity depends solely on amino acid sequence, are the only detectable determinants of collagen.

In the case of globular proteins, our most detailed information available today concerns sperm-whale myoglobin and hen egg-white lysozyme, and these are the only two proteins who will be described in the following, for illustration of this aspect.

Myoglobin is a protein consisting of one polypeptide chain of molecular weight of 18,400, with no disulfide bridges, and containing one heme group per molecule. Large proportion of the molecule (ca. 75%) is arranged in α-helix and β-structure, which maintain the structural integrity of this protein. Immunologically active fragments of myoglobin have been prepared by different procedures such as chymotryptic or tryptic digestion and various techniques for chemical cleavage. The fragments obtained by all the procedure included the same regions of the molecule, which led to the conclusion that in the myoglobin molecule there are 5 antigenically active regions which are separated from each other by antigenically silent areas. These antigenic determinants are located mainly in the non-helical corners at the outer surface of the molecule, and are rather small, consisting of only 6-7 residues (Atassi, 1975), as shown in Figure 2. Examination of a space-filling molecular model of myoglobin reveals that, although the overall shape of the molecule corresponds to a sphere, the surface comprises a series of hillocks and crevices and that the corners of the folded polypeptide chain apparently coincide with some of the more exposed areas. These antigenic determinants, which are confined to definite regions in the molecule that are not helical, are maintained in a fixed rigid conformation by the folding of the molecule. An interesting finding concerning myoglobin is that no definite role can be assigned to any particular residue of the molecule. The residues which participate in the antigenic peptides are those which usually appear on the outer surface of the protein.

Lysozyme, containing several disulfide bonds, which stabilize its structure, is a 'tight' protein and as such is not readily susceptible to proteolysis. Yet, its peptic digestion leads to the formation of two large immunologically active fragments. One of them consists of the two terminal peptides of the molecule, (sequences 1-27 and 122-129), linked together by a disulfide bond (Fujio et al., 1968a, 1968b). The antigenic determinant in this region is as such smaller than the whole fragment, but its exact size has not been determined yet.

The second large fragment consists of the region 57-107, it contains two disulfide bridges and was shown to encompass more than one antigenic determinant. By modifying the digestion conditions this region can yield smaller peptides which are still immunologically active. One of these peptides, comprising residues 60-83, with an intrachain disulfide bond, and denoted 'loop' (Arnon and Sela, 1969), was studied in detail. Its location in the three dimensional structure of lysozyme is shown in Figure 5, and as can be seen, it is exposed on the surface of the molecule. Antibodies specific to this region exclusively, prepared either by selective isolation from anti-lysozyme serum on loop-immuno-adsorbent, or by immunization with a conjugate containing the loop on a synthetic carrier, showed restricted heterogenicity (Maron et al., 1971) and their specificity demonstrated definitely that the loop is a conformation-dependent determinant. The loop antibodies could distinguish between the loop and its open peptide chain and could recognize the loop in the native lysozyme, and consequently react with the intact enzyme.

Lysozyme and myoglobin are just two examples cited here. Many more globular proteins were subjected to a similar type of immunochemical analysis. The results obtained with most of them point to the same conclusion: that globular proteins encompass usually only limited numbers of distinct and independent antigenic determinants, probably four or five. Most of them are on areas of the molecule surface which are more exposed than others, and they usually occupy a rigid and fixed spatial conformation in the three-dimensional structure of the

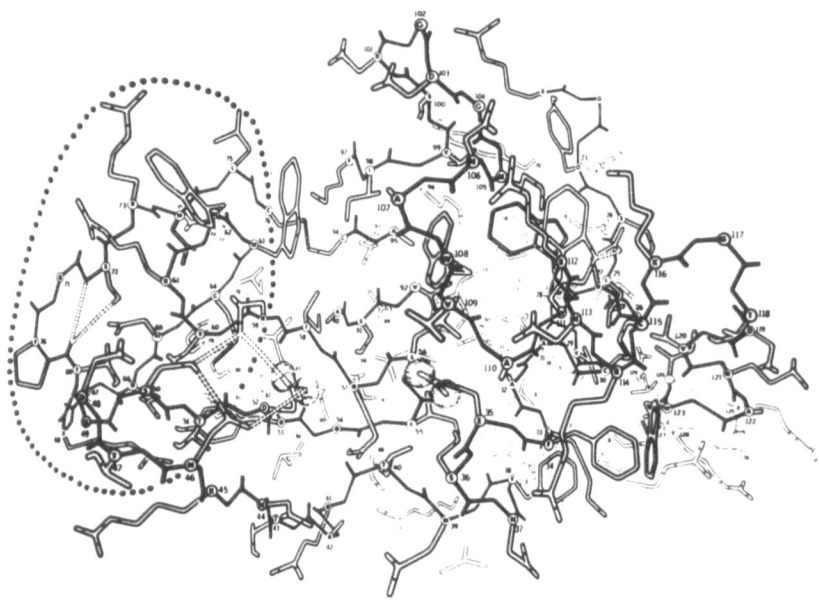

Figure 5

Backbone and side chains of lysozyme. (From Atlas of Protein Sequence and Structure, M. O. Dayhoff, Ed.) The loop region is encircled.

molecule, which is decisive for the antigenic properties. The size of these determinants is rather small (5-7 residues) and is similar in its dimensions to the size of antigenic determinants in polysaccharides and polynucleotides (Kabat, 1968). It is of interest that this size fits very closely the size of the antigen-combining site which was revealed from X-ray crystallography studies of antibody structure (Amzel *et al.*, 1974).

Synthetically Prepared Antigenic Regions of Proteins

The availability of methods for synthesis of peptides with desired sequence on the one hand, and the elucidation of the amino acid sequence of many proteins, including that of defined antigenic regions in them, permitted a synthetic approach to the study of antigenic determinants of native proteins. This approach was proved useful in the investigation of several proteins or polypeptide antigens (reviewed in Arnon, in press). The use of synthetic analogs of a given polypeptide antigenic determinant in which either replacement or a change in size has been introduced, is extremely illuminating as for the role particular residues play in the antigenic specificity of either synthetic or natural antigens.

In the case of the lysozyme molecule and its 'loop' determinant, since the loop region between disulfides Cys_{64} and Cys_{80} is a relatively short peptide segment, consisting of only 17 amino acid residues with a known sequence, it has been feasible to synthesize it, by chemical methods, with the anticipation that the synthetic approach may yield more detailed information regarding the molecular requirements for antigenic specificity. The synthesis was carried out using the solid-phase technique (Merrifield, 1965), yielding a loop-like peptide in which the only difference from the natural loop of lysozyme is the replacement of cysteine in position 76 with alanine, to avoid ambiguous disulfide bond form-ation. The synthesized loop, corresponding to the sequence 64-82 in the amino acid sequence of lysozyme, was identical in its properties and immunological re-activity to the natural loop peptide. Attachment of this peptide to a synthetic carrier (A- -L) resulted in a completely synthetic conjugate which could elicit antibodies reactive with native lysozyme, and still recognizing the conformation-al determinant of the intact molecule (Arnon et al., 1971). Investigation of several synthetic analogs of the loop, in each of which one or two amino acid residues had been replaced by alanine (Teicher et al., 1973), revealed the major role played by particular residues, such as the prolines or the arginines, in the antigenic specificity of this determinant. Moreover, this information was cor-related with the calculated contribution of the various amino acid residues to the β-bends, which constitute the dominant structural feature in this region of lysozyme. A good agreement between the predicted values for the β-bends con-servation and the antigenic reactivity of a particular analog of the loop (Arnon et al., 1974) provided corroberating evidence for the crucial role of the spatial conformation in the specificity of this antigenic determinant.

The use of synthetic ordered peptides have also enabled the preparation of antigens which elicit anti-viral response. Thus, in an early study (Anderer, 1963) it has been shown that the C-terminal hexapeptide of tobacco mosaic virus, when conjugated to a protein carrier, elicited antibodies which reduced to some extent the infectivity of the virus. In a recent study (Langbeheim et al., 1976) we have shown that an effective anti-viral effect can be provoked by a com-pletely synthetic molecule containing an ordered peptide corresponding to a fragment of a virus component.

These studies were carried out with a model system — the MS-2 coliphage. It had previously been reported that the viability of this phage is totally neutral-ized by antiserum prepared against the intact phage. We have shown that this neutralization can, in turn, be inhibited up to 50% by the monomeric form of its coat protein. Furthermore, antiserum prepared by immunization against the isolated coat protein is capable of specifically neutralizing the phage to an extent similar to that obtained with antiphage serum.

In order to locate the region(s) contributing to the neutralizing process, the coat protein was cleaved by CNBr, and the resulting fragments were screened for their inhibitory activity. According to the amino acid sequence of the coat protein (Fig. 6), the expected cleavage at the two methionine residues, 88 and 108, should yield three cleavage products, one of about 10,000 daltons (P_1) and two each of about 2,000 daltons, denoted P_2 and P_3, which indeed was the case. Purified P_1 fragment elicited antiserum which caused 80% neutralization of the phage.

```
Ala - Ser - Asn - Phe - Thr - Gln - Phe - Val - Leu - Val - Asp - Asn - Gly - Gly - Thr - Gly -
                          5                        10                          15
Asp - Val - Thr - Val - Ala - Pro - Ser - Asn - Phe - Ala - Asn - Gly - Val - Ala - Glu - Trp -
                   20                        25                          30
Ile - Ser - Ser - Asn - Ser - Arg - Ser - Gln - Ala - Tyr - Lys - Val - Thr - Cys - Ser - Val -
             35                        40                          45
Arg - Gln - Ser - Ser - Ala - Gln - Asn - Arg - Lys - Tyr - Thr - Ile - Lys - Val - Glu - Val -
       50                        55                          60
Pro - Lys - Val - Ala - Thr - Gln - Thr - Val - Gly - Gly - Val - Glu - Leu - Pro - Val - Ala -
 65                        70                        75                          80
Ala - Trp - Arg - Ser - Tyr - Leu - Asn - Met - Glu - Leu - Thr - Ile - Pro - Ile - Phe - Ala -
                   85                        90                          95
Thr - Asn - Ser - Asp - Cys - Glu - Leu - Ile - Val - Lys - Ala - Met - Gln - Gly - Leu - Leu -
                  100                        105                         110
Lys - Asp - Gly - Asn - Pro - Ile - Pro - Ser - Ala - Ile - Ala - Ala - Asn - Ser - Gly - Ile - Tyr
            115                        120                          125
```

Figure 6

Sequence of bacteriophage MS-2 coat-protein. The arrows indicate the points of cleavage by cyanogen bromide at methionine residues 88 and 108.

The mixture of the two small fragments, P_2 and P_3, was capable of inhibiting the neutralization of the MS-2 phage by whole anti-phage serum, as depicted in Figure 7. The extent of inhibition was almost 40%, close to the value obtained with the intact coat protein. Efforts to separate the fragments P_2 and P_3 from the mixture failed due to the negligible difference in their molecular size and their almost equal net electrical charge. To determine which of the two small fragments described above shows the inhibitory effect on the phage neutralization, synthesis was attempted, by the solid phase technique (Arnon *et al.*, 1971) of the two peptides corresponding in sequence to fragments P_2 and P_3, and both were evaluated for their capacity to inhibit the neutralization of MS-2 by the whole anti-phage serum. In contrast to P_3, which did not exhibit any inhibitory activity, the synthetic P_2 possessed high inhibitory activity, almost identical to the inhibition effected by a similar concentration of the mixture of the P_2 and P_3 fragments obtained by cleavage of the native coat protein.

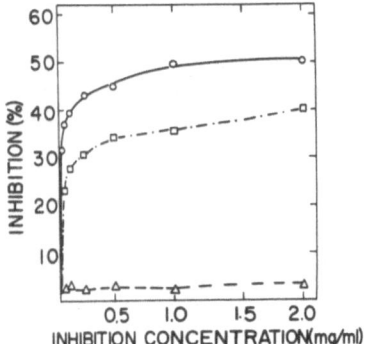

Figure 7

Inhibition of MS-2 phage neutralization by anti-phage antiserum (dilution 3×10^{-4}) with intact MS-2 coat-protein (o——o), mixture of the native peptides P_2 and P_3 (□ — · — □) and phosphate buffer control (△----△).

Conjugates of the two peptides attached to the synthetic carrier A- -L served for immunization of rabbits and the resultant antisera were tested for their capacity to neutralize MS-2 phage. As shown in Figure 8, while anti P_3-A- -L showed essentially no neutralizing activity, the antiserum against P_2-A- -L had neutralizing capacity to an extent of 85%, comparable with that obtained by the anti-coat protein.

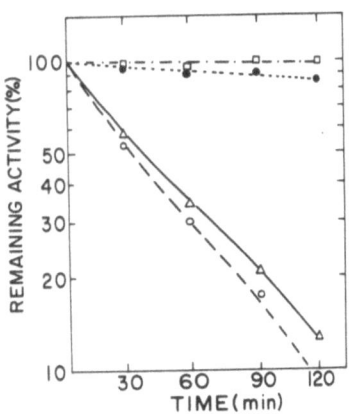

Figure 8

Neutralization of MS-2 phage by various antisera: anti-coat-protein serum (dilution 10^{-3}) (o---o); anti P_2-A- -L serum (dilution 3×10^{-3}) (△——△); anti P_3-A- -L serum (dilution 3×10^{-3}) (●---●); normal rabbit serum (dilution 10^{-3}) (□-----□).

We have thus demonstrated that a completely synthetic antigen can be used for induction of an immune response resulting in the phage neutralization. This may serve as an additional step in the direction of synthetic vaccines, a possibility in a remote future.

Concluding Remarks

The use of synthetic materials in the field of vaccination against viruses may be envisaged to have several advantages over the use of intact, attenuated or killed viruses. First, theoretically it should be possible to attach several peptides, representing the relevant portions of different viruses, to the same carrier molecule. Thus, each adequately designed synthetic antigen will be multivalent, and capable to replace several narrowly specific vaccines. Second, this approach might eliminate immunization against many irrelevant antigenic determinants of the virus, or of irrelevant proteins which contaminate the viral preparation used for vaccination. Thus, frequently occurring undesired side-reactions may be avoided. Third, for many vaccines, the addition of an adjuvant is required in order to initiate an immune response; some of these adjuvants are not suitable for human use. In a synthetic macromolecule this problem of adjuvanticity may find its solution by introduction of certain groups which enhance antigenicity. Antigens so designed may possess built-in adjuvanticity and may prove of less hazard.

The prerequisite for preparation of a synthetic vaccine is the availability of an immunologically active fragment which is involved in the neutralization process and hence has a chance of evoking neutralizing antibodies. For this purpose, it is essential to obtain more information on the chemistry of antigenic determinants and to elucidate their contribution to the manifold manifestation of immunity.

REFERENCES

AMZEL, L. M., POLJAK, R. J., SAUL, F., VARGA, J. M. and RICHARDS, F. F. (1974) Proc. Nat. Acad. Sci. 71, 1427-1430.
ANDERER, F. A. (1963) Biochim. Biophys. Acta 71, 246-248.
ARNON, R. (1977) in 'Immunochemistry' (Glynn, ed.) John Wiley, N.Y. in press.
ARNON, R. and MARON, E. (1970) J. Mol. Biol. 51, 703-707.
ARNON, R. and MARON, E. (1971) J. Mol. Biol. 61, 225-235.
ARNON, R., MARON, E., SELA, M. and ANFINSEN, C. B. (1971) Proc. Nat. Acad. Sci. 68, 1450-1455.
ARNON, R. and SELA, M. (1960) Biochem. J. 75, 103-109.
ARNON, R. and SELA, M. (1969) Proc. Nat. Acad. Sci. 62, 163-170.
ARNON, R., TEICHER, E. and SCHERAGA, H. A. (1974) J. Mol. Biol. 90, 403-407.
ATASSI, M. Z. (1975) Immunochemistry 12, 423-438.
BECKER, U., TIMPL, R. and KULIN, K. (1972) Eur. J. Biochem. 28, 221-231.

BREW, K., CASTELLINO, F. J., VANAMAN, T. C., TRAYER, I. P. and MATTOCK, P. (1969) Brookhaven Symp. Biol. No. 21, Vol. 1, pp. 139.

CEBRA, J. J. (1961) J. Immunol. *86*, 190-196; 205-214.

CRUMPTON, M. J. (1974) in 'The Antigens' (Sela, M., ed.) Vol. II, pp.1, Academic Press, New York.

CRUMPTON, M. J. and WILKINSON, J. M. (1966) Biochem. J. *100*, 223-232.

DICKERSON, R. E. (1964) in 'The Proteins' (Neurath, H., ed.) 2nd ed., Vol. II, pp. 603, Academic Press, New York.

FUCHS, S. and SELA, M. (1963) Biochem. J. *87*, 70-79.

FUJIO, H., IMANISHI, M., NISHIOKA, K. and AMANO, T. (1968a) Biken J. *11*, 207-218.

FUJIO, H., IMANISHI, M., NISHIOKA, K. and AMANO, T. (1968b) Biken J. *11*, 219-223.

KABAT, E. A. (1968) in 'Structural Concepts in Immunology and Immunochemistry' pp.89, Holt, Rinehart and Winston Inc. New York.

LANGBEHEIM, H., ARNON. R. and SELA, M. (1976) Proc. Nat. Acad. Sci. *73*, 4636-4640.

LAPRESLE, C. and DARIEUX, J. (1957) Ann. Inst. Pasteur *92*, 62.

MARON, E., SHIOZAWA, C., ARNON, R. and SELA, M. (1971) Biochemistry *10*, 763-771.

MERRIFIELD, R. B. (1965) Science *150*, 178-185.

MOZES, E., SCHWARTZ, M. and SELA, M. (1974) J. Exp. Med. *140*, 349-355.

PORTER, R. P. (1957) Biochem. J. *66*, 677-686.

SCHECHTER, B., SCHECHTER, I., RAMACHANDRAN, J., CONWAY-JACOBS, A., SELA, M., BENJAMIN, E. and SHIMIZU, M. (1971) Eur. J. Biochem. *20*, 309-320.

SELA, M. and ARNON, R. (1960a) Biochem. J. *75*, 91-102.

SELA, M. and ARNON, R. (1960b) Biochem. J. *77*, 394-399.

SELA, M. and ARNON, R. (1960c) Biochim. Biophys. Acta *40*, 382-384.

SELA, M., FUCHS, S. and ARNON, R. (1962) Biochem. J. *85*, 223-235.

SELA, M. and MOZES, E. (1966) Proc. Nat. Acad. Sci. *55*, 445-452.

SELA, M., SCHECHTER, B., SCHECHTER, I. and BOREK, F. (1967) Cold Spring Harbor Symp. Quant. Biol. *32*, 537-545.

TEICHER, E., MARON, E. and ARNON, R. (1973) Immunochemistry *10*, 265-271.

DE WECK, A. L. (1974) in 'The Antigens' (Sela, M., ed.) Vol. II, pp. 141, Academic Press, New York.

LIST OF PARTICIPANTS

Dr. Ruth Arnon
    Department of Chemical Immunology,
    The Weizmann Institute of Science,
    Rehovot,
    Israel.

Dr. Gillian Air
    Department of Microbiology,
    John Curtin School of Medical Research,
    Austrailian National University,
    P. O. Box 334,
    Canberra City,   A.C.T. 2601
    Australia.

Dr. Helmut Bachmayer
    Sandoz Forschungsinstitut,
    A-1235 Wien,
    Brunner Strasse 59,
    Austria.

Ms Elaine Brown
    Division of Biophysics,
    National Institute for Medical Research,
    Mill Hill,
    London,   NW7 1AA
    England.

Dr. Doris Bucher
    Department of Microbiology,
    Mount Sinai School of Medicine
    of the City University of New York,
    Fifth Avenue and 100th Street,
    New York,
    N.Y. 10021, USA.

Dr. Purnell Choppin
    The Rockefeller University,
    1230 York Avenue,
    New York,
    N.Y. 10021, USA.

Dr. Stephen Fazekas de St. Groth
C.S.I.R.O.,
Genetics Research Laboratories,
Molecular and Cellular Biology Unit,
P. O. Box 90,
Epping,
N.S.W. 2121
Australia.

Dr. Walter Gerhard
Wistar Institute,
36th and Spruce Streets,
Philadelphia,
Pa 19104, USA.

Dr. Mary Jane Gething
Imperial Cancer Research Fund,
Lincoln's Inn Fields,
London,   WC2A 3PX
England.

Dr. Hans-Dieter Klenk
Institut für Virologie,
Justus Liebig Universität,
6300 Giessen,
Frankfurter Strasse 107,
Germany.

Dr. Christian Kunz
Institut für Virologie der Universität Wien,
Kinderspitalgasse 15,
A-1090 Wien,
Austria.

Dr. R. LaMontagne
Department of Health Education and Welfare,
Public Health Service,
National Institutes of Health,
Building 31A, Room 7A10,
Bethesda,
Md. 20014, USA.

Dr. W. Graeme Laver
    Department of Microbiology,
    John Curtin School of Medical Research,
    Australian National University,
    P. O. Box 334,
    Canberra City, A.C.T. 2601
    Australia.

Dr. Ekke Liehl
    Sandoz Forschungsinstitut,
    A-1235 Wien,
    Brunner Strasse 59,
    Austria.

Dr. John McCauley
    Imperial Cancer Research Fund,
    Lincoln's Inn Fields,
    London,   WC2A 3PX
    England.

Dr. Bernie Moss
    C.S.I.R.O.,
    Genetics Research Laboratories,
    Molecular and Cellular Biology Unit,
    P. O. Box 90,
    Epping,
    N.S.W. 2121
    Australia.

Dr. Brian Murphy
    Laboratory of Infectious Diseases,
    National Institute of Allergy and Infectious Diseases,
    National Institutes of Health,
    Public Health Service,
    Department of Health Education and Welfare,
    Bethesda,
    Md. 20014, USA.

Dr. Y. Nakashima
    Imperial Cancer Research Fund,
    Lincoln's Inn Fields,
    London,   WC2A 3PX
    England.

Dr. Peter Palese
    Department of Microbiology,
    Mount Sinai School of Medicine
    of the City University of New York,
    Fifth Avenue and 100th Street,
    New York,
    N.Y. 10029, USA.

Dr. Peter Reeve
    Sandoz Forschungsinstitut
    A-1235 Wien,
    Brunner Strasse 59,
    Austria.

Dr. Rudolf Rott
    Institut für Virologie,
    Justus Liebig Universität,
    6300 Giessen,
    Frankfurter Strasse 107,
    Germany.

Dr. John Skehel
    World Influenza Center,
    National Institute for Medical Research,
    Mill Hill,
    London,   NW7 1AA
    England.

Dr. Geoffrey C. Schild
    Head, Division of Viral Products,
    National Institute for Biological Standards and Control,
    London,   NW3 6RB
    England.

Dr. Christoph Scholtissek
    Institut für Virologie,
    Justus Liebig Universität,
    6300 Giessen,
    Frankfurter Strasse 107,
    Germany.

Dr. Irene Schulze
Department of Microbiology,
St. Louis University School of Medicine,
1042 South Grand Boulevard,
St. Louis,
Mo. 63104, USA.

Dr. Colin Ward
C.S.I.R.O.,
Division of Protein Chemistry,
343 Royal Parade,
Parkville,
Victoria 3052
Australia.

Dr. Mike Waterfield
Imperial Cancer Research Fund,
Lincoln's Inn Fields,
London,   WC2A 3PX
England.

Dr. Robert G. Webster
St. Jude Children's Research Hospital,
P. O. Box 318,
Memphis,
Tenn. 38101, USA.

Dr. Rudolf Weil
Sandoz Forschungsinstitut,
A-1235 Wien,
Brunner Strasse 59,
Austria.

Dr. Donald C. Wiley
Chemistry Department,
Harvard University,
12 Oxford Street,
Cambridge,
Mass. 02138, USA.

Dr. Nicholas G. Wrigley
Division of Biophysics,
National Institute for Medical Research,
Mill Hill,
London,   NW7 1AA, England.

LIST OF AUTHORS

A

- at rough endoplasmatic reticulum; 91
- at smooth endoplasmatic
reticulum; 91

H

HA, light and heavy chains;
69, 70, 72, 83, 141, 149, 152-
164, 168, 204-206
-, ----, separation on Bio-
gel P150;149, 152-
154
-, preparation of, using
bromelain; 131, 132, 136-
138, 148, 150, 168
-,--, using SDS; 122, 141,
168, 203-205
-,--, using Brij 36T; 133,
135
HA_0; 93
Haem group; 229, 230, 231
Hemagglutination inhibitors;
112, 114
Herd immunity; 39, 47
Hierarchic series (Hierarchy)
see also hierarchic mutants;
158-164
HN from Sendai virus; 215,
216, 221
Hydrophilic end of influenza
hemagglutinin; 13
Hydrophobic peptide; 133, 135,
137, 138, 190-191
-- Sendai F-protein; 222

I

Immunogenicity of proteins
and synthetic polypeptides;
225-240
Influenza B virus, see Influ-
enza virus strains
Influenza Virus Strains
HON1
A/Bellamy/42; 15-20, 141-144,
183, 195, 196-198
A/BH/35; 15-21

A/Hickcox/40; 15-21
A/Melbourne/35; 15, 16, 18-21,
140,
A/PR/8/34; 6, 15-19, 21-23,
40-46, 50, 51, 61, 63, 65-67,
71, 80, 140, 146, 203
A/WS/33; 63, 65, 66
A/WSE/33; 15-21
A/WSN/33; 51, 52, 54, 76, 104,
195
A/Weiss/43; 15-20, 131, 140
H1N1
A/CAM/46; 15-20, 40-44
A/FM/1/47; 8, 15-20, 61, 63,
65, 66. 71, 80, 140-144
H2N2
A/Nederland/84/68; 140-144
A/Japan/305/57; 133, 134, 139,
167-179, 181-189
A/Singapore/57; 40-43, 61, 66,
67, 71, 80
H3N2
A/Aichi/68; 36, 37
A/ART/74; 38
A/England/845/69; 35-37
A/England/878/69; 35, 37
A/England/42/72; 35, 37, 203
A/DEC/71; 37
A/Finland/74; 38, 39
A/Hong Kong/68; 4-10, 12, 23,
33, 50, 51, 61, 65, 66, 80,
131, 203
A/Hong Kong/107/71; 36, 37
A/Hannover/74; 38, 39
A/LAS/71; 35, 37
A/Memphis/102/72; 2-6, 121-
125, 193-201
A/NG/75; 38
A/North Territory/60/68; 33,
35, 37, 38, 40-43, 146, 151,
153-164
A/Port Chalmers/73; 2, 4, 6-8,
10, 38, 39
A/PR/1/73; 35, 37
A/PR/2/74; 38, 39
A/Scotland/840/74; 9, 12, 38
A/Victoria/3/75; 38, 39, 141-
144
A/Victoria/112/76; 38, 39

X

Z

———————